Commissioning Domiciliary Care

A practical guide to purchasing services

Colleen Rothwell-Murray

Foreword by
Sir Sandy Macara

Radcliffe Medical Press Ltd
18 Marcham Road, Abingdon, Oxon OX14 1AA

This book has been written to increase the understanding within the health and social services professions, and others about the subject. While every effort has been made to ensure its accuracy, it does not set out to be a legal guide, and the author, publisher, distributor and retailer cannot be held liable to any person or entity for losses caused or alleged to be caused by reliance on this book.

British Library Cataloguing in Publication Data

A catalogue record for this book is available from the British Library.

ISBN 1 85775 333 X

Typeset by Action Publishing Technology Ltd, Gloucester
Printed and bound by Biddles Ltd, Guildford and King's Lynn

Contents

Foreword

'Hast thou no care of me?' How many frail elderly, mentally ill or disabled people in the UK today echo Cleopatra's anguished cry?

Over 50 years ago, when the Welfare State was introduced, the sound-bite was 'freedom from fear'. Put more positively, the assurance through insurance and taxation was of care in relation to need 'from the cradle to the grave'. Demography and costs have combined to cheat the young inheritors of that expectation. Too many of us now live too long for personal or physical comfort. The cost of care – whether physical, mental or social – has soared beyond that of general inflation and the capacity of a lifetime's hard-earned savings to provide even for the most provident individual.

But surely the state was going to provide a safety net? In practice, the National Health Service (NHS), chronically underfunded relative to other comparable healthcare systems, finds domiciliary care increasingly difficult to fund and regards institutional care – other than in hospital – as the responsibility of the social services. Social service departments are similarly strapped for funds due to capping of local government expenditure. Hence the imposition of means testing for both institutional care and for domiciliary social services. This depressing scene is curiously in conflict with the contemporary concern to promote individual rights through much vaunted patients' charters and political manifestos. Politicians of every hue claim that the tax-paying community as a whole is not prepared to vote for additional resources: sadly, they are probably right. Hence the imperative of making the best use of all the existing resources, including those available to individuals in their own homes. Support to family and other voluntary carers is therefore crucial because most people rightly choose to remain in familiar surroundings for as long as humanly possible.

The report of the Royal Commission on the Care of the Elderly, published on 1 March 1999, seeks to make a distinction between healthcare, which should be provided by the NHS, and social care, which should be provided by social service departments. This questionable distinction will clearly be the subject of fervid debate; meanwhile, everyone concerned has to get on with the job. Colleen Rothwell-Murray's guide meets an urgent and continuing need for clear, straightforward advice for those professionally responsible for the provision of domiciliary care. It is refreshingly free of the kind of jargon which too often bedevils books of this kind, nor does it try to do too much; references are provided for those who need fuller information. However, the spectrum of cover is commendably wide, encompassing every essential aspect of the structure and function of services, including such vital aspects of care as quality, continuity, privacy and indemnity.

Sir Sandy Macara
July 1999

About the author

Colleen Rothwell-Murray has worked in healthcare and social services for 16 years, and until recently managed a domiciliary care provider unit. After graduating as a mature student in Law, she was a further education lecturer and now works for BMA Regional Services.

This book is dedicated to my family, Christopher, Daisy and Alastair, without whose help and support this enterprise could not have been undertaken.

List of abbreviations

ADLs	Activities of Daily Living
CCS	Commission for Care Standards
CPA	Continuing Power of Attorney
EAA	Employment Agencies Act
EPA	Enduring Power of Attorney
FRES	Federation of Recruitment and Employment Services
GMS	general medical services
GSCC	General Social Care Council
HA	health authority
HSC	Health and Safety Commission
HSE	Health and Safety Executive
HSWA	Health and Safety at Work, etc. Act 1974
MRSA	methicillin-resistant *Staphylococcus aureus*
NA	nursing auxiliaries
NCVO	National Council for Voluntary Organisations
NHS	National Health Service
NHST	National Health Service Trust
NVQ	National Vocational Qualification
PIA	Personal Investment Authority
PIN	personal identification number
RCN	Royal College of Nursing
SSD	Social Services Department
UKCC	United Kingdom Central Council for Nurses and Midwives
UKHCA	United Kingdom Homecare Association
WTD	Working Time Directive

Introduction

This book stems from the basis of the expansion in requirements for care, the relative high costs of private residential and nursing homes, and the potential consequences for occupational rights for home owners. The preamble is the contraction of the NHS services in 'geriatric' medicine, together with the prevailing negative views on the traditional institutionalised methods of care. The recent fashion on individual rights, patients' charter and the enshrined rights of disabled people in statute have meant that the demand for 'care ' to be provided at home is growing. But non-healthcare is not freely available, and has not been hitherto. At this level of home care, which is not classified by an earlier Secretary of State for Health as healthcare, availability of, or access to, the service may be detached from the issues of quality and cost. In this debate, choice has been promoted as an empowering concept.

In this book, 'commissioning' is the term used for converting the process of 'delivery of care' into a business mechanism, where there are buyers, sellers, products and outcomes. The overall business term is 'purchasing', a vital theme which is a core activity in all producers of goods. But within the service sector, which includes health and social services, the principles of purchasing are less well understood.

The book has been written for those health- and social-care professionals who either have the task of purchasing domiciliary care or of advising on its suitability for adults. It is anticipated that an ever-increasing number of professional people will require an adequate understanding of the principles of purchasing and the ethics related to delivering care in order to provide a quality service in their field of work, whether or not it is in the health- or social-care arenas. There are major disputes about what constitutes care at home, and this book does not address that debate, but rather, it highlights problem areas where a controlling professional will need a level of awareness in determining the suitability of the care systems available.

It will not apply to the care provisions for children. It is not an academic text for theorists and students of care provision, neither is it a law book in the traditional sense, but the references will assist those who need to have more detailed background information.

Not only is purchasing care a hugely expanding activity,[1] but purchasing is becoming a more usual method of obtaining services,[2] and even where services are provided within an organisation, purchasing principles are utilised as a measuring tool. The developments in primary care have adopted the principles recently exploited in the total purchasing of healthcare services. The imminence of the 'arranged marriage' between health and social care, spelled out in the consultation paper *Partnership in Action* will demand closer joint working between health and social services; 'The overhaul is long overdue. Endless hours have been spent arguing over when someone living at home who need assistance with bathing is a "health" or a "social" bath case'.[3]

Legal jargon is avoided where possible, to increase the accessibility of the book to professionals who have not had any formal legal training. But legal principles are explored, and it is essential for professionals to grasp their relevance in understanding how these services are delivered.

References, provided at the end of each chapter, will give pointers to those who need to research a topic more fully. Domiciliary care will be defined as 'help with social and domestic tasks such as cleaning, washing and preparing meals, with disablement equipment and home adaptations, transport, budgeting and other aspects of daily living'.[4]

The NHS and Community Care Act 1990 provided for the basic rights of individual citizens to choose to be cared for within their own homes. The White Paper, *Caring for People: Community Care in the Next Decade and Beyond*, gives the detailed reasoning behind the decisions to provide care in this way, and the reasons for reducing the number of people residing in local authority residential homes.

Very few argue that this domiciliary approach is unwanted or unreasonable. But it is important to realise that social services are a means-tested benefit, and so tend to be concentrated within a sector of the population. Furthermore, the delivery of services to the homes of individuals must be a realistic option for the organisations designated to ensure the fulfilment of the goals set out in the White Paper.

The lead agency for undertaking community care assessments is the Social Services Department (SSD) within local government. There have been a series of court cases in the past 5 years, challenging the decision of the local SSD to withdraw, reduce or limit community care services. In a recent decision of the Court of Appeal, the judgement, *R v. Bristol City Council ex parte* Penfold [1998] 1 CCLR 315 QPB, indicates that the duties of SSDs to be informed of the needs of their local populations is extant, even if the SSD is unable to provide any service. Entitlement to community care, then, is a highly contentious debate.

Like any new health- or social-care activity, it is vital that the highest standards are met in relation to access, quality and costs. Newspapers abound with horror stories of poor health services, especially where the patients or clients are classified as vulnerable; 'The expansion of unregulated domiciliary services therefore remains a worrying development given that they are provided to some of the most vulnerable and isolated members of our communities in the privacy of their own homes'.[5]

Unlike providing nursing care, where the managers can have a degree of confidence in the skills of the nursing staff, this non-nursing care is not governed by any specific authority, and the organisations who provide private care are not compelled to work to any specific standards. This creates a void of uncertainty, which the Secretary of State for Health, Mr Frank Dobson, has acknowledged, and promised to address in the not too distant future.

The lack of regulation can lead to uncertainty about standards of care. The ideal situation is that after the parties to a bargain have decided what the contract is about (there should be no debate about the desired outcome), an agreement, including the price, can be reached. In cases of care contracting, it may be more desirable to state outcomes. However, it seems to be more common that specifications are stated. This is less clear when the service is not standardised, and people who have purchased 'care' are not content with the service. Where the recipient of the service is not the purchaser, getting to grips with the specifications can be even more difficult. For whom are the standards? The majority of organisations delivering a service aim to satisfy the 'customer', otherwise known as the one who pays.

References

1 LeGrand J, Mays N and Mulligan J-A (eds) (1998) *Learning from the Internal Market: a review of the evidence.* King's Fund, London.

2 Harden I (1992) *The Contracting State.* Open University Press, Buckingham.

3 Eaton L (1998) Arranged marriages. *Health Service J.* **108**: 24.

4 Department of Health and Social Security (1989) *Caring for People: Community Care in the Next Decade and Beyond*, Cmd. 849, para. 2.4. HMSO, London.

5 Griffiths A and Roberts G (eds) (1995) *The Law and Elderly People*, p. 135. Routledge, London.

1
The nature of purchasing

Purchasing is the public service word for buying or contracting in the course of their business. Large organisations such as civil service departments, local authorities and the NHS, as well as commercial firms, obtain goods and services from outside sources.

This is different from commissioning, which is the word reserved for internal exchanges or 'contracts', within an organisation, which mimic the free market. Many public organisations now regard some of their departments or functions as separate organisations, and the transactions between them are conducted as if the departments were commercial firms. This general trend of 'privatisation' has suffered from a degree of unpopularity in the eyes of some of the staff inside the organisations, as well as external commentators.

Nevertheless, those involved in commissioning who previously had more of an administrative role have had to familiarise themselves with market behaviour, and there is a growing acknowledgement of the need for ethical purchasing practices.

An essential feature in successful commissioning is the necessity to know the 'partners' of the commissioning process, to understand their values and expectations. In the NHS commissioning process, there is a recognition of the need for transparency in the communications between 'purchaser and supplier'. Such transparency is not the generality in commercial purchasing, and in fact is directly contrary to the rules in local authority compulsory competitive tendering.

However, prior to the 'privatisation' trend, local authorities commonly contracted with commercial firms to provide services, and building contracts for the 'local council' were generally sought after in the local business fraternity. The Local Government Planning and Land Act 1980 provided for compulsory competitive tendering with respect to construction and maintenance work, which meant that outside commercial contractors had to tender for this type of work, competing all the while with the 'in-house' council department. In 1988, the Local

Government Act extended the number of activities that had to be 'contracted' in this way.

The methodology adopted in the range of private and public organisations in purchasing is enormous. Tendering may not be the only method of enlisting suppliers.

Generally, within each department various members of staff who are authorised to make such decisions as to which other companies or organisations to deal with, act as agents for the purchasing company, and will make contact with similarly placed agents of the reciprocating company. Thus, both organisations will be 'legal personalities', such as a limited company, a public limited company or a statutory corporation such as a local authority or a health authority or a National Health Service Trust (NHST). These organisations have complex internal structures, and various levels within the structures will deal with separate components of the purchase, such as terms and conditions of trading, billing and finance, quality control and so forth.

Departmental staff may inherit from a departed predecessor a list of contractors to purchase from, or there may be periodic reviews or short-term contracts determined by tenders. This kind of purchasing is a specialised field of study, and those who take it up are often required to have qualifications from institutes such as the Chartered Institute of Purchasing and Supplies.

Generally, a member of staff, from any firm, who has ascertained that goods or services are required for the job in hand, will need to confirm this with a superior – a line manager perhaps – and then complete a form usually called a requisition, which is sent to a central department. That department would then place a purchase order on the supplier to provide the goods or services. It could be a standard category of goods (e.g. bricks from a builders' merchant) or a non-standard load (e.g. tons of a special mix of concrete for a unique statue).

The complexity and formality of this basic process varies according to the nature of the product or service and the requirement for evaluation of need and supplier, and the need for definition, economy and control. The four key stages in this process are:

1 recognition/initiation of need

2 supplier selection

3 placing of purchase order, i.e. instruction to supply

4 supply of goods or services.

These stages are subject to an enormous variability in their implementation, from the very informal verbal to the highly formal involving many people, reports and meetings. Timescales, equally, vary from very short to very long. The process depends on the complexity, novelty and intervals of the goods or services in question. The technical evaluation of goods is more easily accomplished than for services, especially where the need for economy dominates the thought processes.

Buying or purchasing goods in the course of business is a highly skilled and complex activity, with many possible pitfalls for the untrained. Advertising for suppliers to tender is fairly common. This amounts to an invitation for such suppliers to make a tentative or firm offer of such goods or services. The formation and submission of such 'bids' usually take a particular form, depending on the type of market sector.

The basic common law rules of contract will apply. The offeree accepts the terms of the offeror of the goods or services and pays the price or consideration. Both parties must have the intention to create legal relations, have the capacity to contract and any representations made to induce the contract must be valid. There should be no mistakes, no undue influence, no duress and the Unfair Contract Terms Act 1977 provides grounds for a contracting party to object to onerous or oppressive terms in a contract. The contract must be legal, and there is a vast array of restrictions that the courts have held to be unlawful.

Each organisation must set out the rules under which it will operate and ensure that when a contract is created, any foreseeable losses that might arise are borne by the sellers. The drafting of legal documents to support the contract, which may be used in litigation or commercial arbitration, is often undertaken by staff who are legally qualified.

Any goods being purchased would be purchased with the terms and conditions that favour the purchasing organisation and not the other side – the sellers. An example of this type of rule is the date at which the goods are accepted, signifying the moment when ownership from the seller is transferred to the buyer. Where the transaction relates to valuable commodities, insurance of the goods will be crucial, and if the goods are damaged, the insurers will want to know the precise moment when ownership in the goods was transferred. These terms and conditions – often known as the small print – are generally printed on the purchaser's official documentation at the time of bidding; the potential supplier will have included in the quotation their own terms and conditions, e.g. when payment is due. Sometimes negotiation takes place to vary the other party's terms and conditions (e.g. the supplier wants payment in 30 days, but the purchaser wants 60 days). The mismatch between the buyer's and seller's terms can be critical. Many court cases are called to determine the meaning of these terms and conditions.[a]

Purchasing services can be even more complex, because the purchaser might have to define in much more detail, the components, quality and pricing of the service. An example might be the alteration or repair of plumbing in an office or workplace. Choosing a supplier of the service can be difficult if the purchaser does not regularly use such a service. The example of a plumber will be used to demonstrate the gap between purchaser and supplier. The purchaser must then define what the plumber must do – and both purchaser and plumber might have different ideas about the job, because the skilled tradesman might have more knowledge of the kind of problems affecting the repair than the purchaser.

Frequently, in a large organisation, the member of staff who knows a good deal about the work required will outline the job for the plumber and the finance department will agree to pay the plumber on the basis that some senior member of staff has stipulated clearly the description of the work and its price. Thus, in a hospital, there may be an estates department which looks after the land and buildings, and will deal with plumbers, electricians, builders and so forth. There may be a standardised way in which such relationships are dealt with, and the plumber will be informed that the specifications, dates, method of payment, etc. will be according to the organisation's systems. Payment may be conditional on a completion certificate which must be signed by the relevant member of staff and which will then 'trigger' the payment process.

But in smaller organisations, there are fewer skilled staff with different types of skills. A bakery, for example, which employs a dozen people will not have staff dedicated to a single aspect of the organisation, and when a service is sought, such as a plumbing repair or the installation of a computer system, it is likely that the senior staff will have to exercise skills over a wider range of activities. It is very likely that in such a case, where there is an 'information asymmetry', an inevitable degree of dependence will occur – where the bakery owner depends on what the plumber or systems analyst says about the job to be done. In cases such as these there is, inevitably, a transfer of power from the purchaser to the seller. The seller has to be trusted not to 'overquote', by selling services that the purchaser does not need. There are many examples of this

[a]*Butler Machine Tool Company Ltd v. Ex-Cell-O Corporation* [1979] 1 All ER 965 is an example of the difficulties in establishing whose terms and conditions applied to the transaction, which involved a variation in price clause. In order for this clause to be applied, the terms and conditions would have to be those of the party wishing to assert the clause. So, the question was, on whose terms was the transaction effected?

unethical practice, the mis-selling of personal pensions to people who are already members of an adequate occupational pension scheme being a typical example.

The problems endured by purchasers, then, are centred around definition and control. Not only must they find the right supplier, but they must then ensure that the goods match the required specifications. Controlling the nature, choice, price, delivery, quality and timing of the goods and services will be an overriding concern. The ability to control depends upon knowledge, and the amount of effort deployed to understand all that is required, including the variety of suppliers and the effort of monitoring the supply itself.

Purchasing goods – historically the preponderant type of purchase – has required the inclusion of details and specifications. Goods bought often have to be put to use with other goods. The physical details are of profound significance to engineers, technicians and the like. But contracts for standard services rarely need to include much in the way of detail with regard to how the service is delivered. If booking a surgical operation or ordering a conveyance on your house are used as examples, the trend is that the document referring to the contractual undertakings, if there is one, is short. Outcomes may be specified.

Purchasers understand and recognise the 'outcomes' for services such as accountancy, conveyancing, will writing, house contents removal, household repairs, appliance repairs and so forth. The purpose of the contract for services in the majority of cases is obvious. A failure to achieve the outcome is also usually transparent.

The nature of selling

Most commercial organisations are in the business of selling their products or services, which are designed to meet a specific market demand. Thus, manufacturers of confectionery will market their product through advertising, special offers or promotions, etc. to maximise the number of sales. Solicitors advertise their services in the newspapers, specialised press, Yellow Pages, commercial radio, give talks to the public, meet heads of business organisations and so forth to maximise the number of fee-paying clients or the fees the clients pay.

New markets are constantly developing, and at the initial phase, when the demand is established, there is likely to be a shortage or undersupply (e.g. mobile telephones in the late 1980s), but as soon as the extent of the demand is anticipated, the market becomes saturated with the product. Each seller must then define clearly for themselves which market sectors are relevant to them and scale their marketing activity accordingly.

Marketing, then, is the central feature of the sellers, requiring great attention to product, placing, pricing and promotion, all of which will be affected by competitors as well as purchasers.

The nature of selling healthcare services

Healthcare is notoriously undersupplied – that is to say, many more people want healthcare than the suppliers of healthcare can provide. In the UK National Health Service, this demand is regulated by the government, who provide healthcare on a conditional basis. Each citizen is entitled to be on the list of a general practitioner, and the GP will decide what NHS services a patient can have. The GP acts as the gateway to the 'market' of health services, and once a patient has entered within it, the internal market in healthcare is the mechanism through which it is supplied. The patient is not a party to this internal market, but can be regarded as a beneficiary of the system. If a patient wants to buy private healthcare, then the criterion is usually affordability, but can also be an undersupply of the market.

Complementary therapies, which can be available free through some GPs, can be bought privately, but are not necessarily always available in the buyer's location. There are enormous problems here related to definitions, outcomes, standardisation and quality.[1] No figures are available as to the profitability of these services, but supply is becoming much more plentiful.

Most private orthodox medical care is bought through private medical insurance policies by individuals or consumers. Thus, the 'product' that is being marketed here is not the healthcare itself, but a financial product; that is to say, a bet or a gamble that the consumer will never require the healthcare which is portrayed so generously. The actual cost of such healthcare services is rarely referred to in advertising such services.

The central theme of selling healthcare services then, relates to its availability, intimately related to its price. Those in a position to sell, such as the private hospitals, must sell at certain minimum prices which reflect the skill of the workers providing the service. In high-skill occupations, the workers will only work for high wages, or perhaps more properly, large fees.

The nature of purchasing healthcare services

The organisations that purchase private healthcare in the UK tend to be large organisations that provide occupational health services for their staff. Organisations undertaking high-risk activities (such as nuclear power production, mining, deep sea exploration, etc.) tend to have an occupational health department or use an external occupational health physician. Nowadays, prisons, borstals, private schools, nursing homes and firms contract for a provider of such medical services, and the process is fairly standardised.

The role of the GP, providing what is known as general medical services (GMS), is well established in the UK, and many 'private' organisations use this as a model for developing their own service. Contracting for GPs by the government has become a fairly standardised process. The model for purchasing healthcare can be found in the way the Department of Health, through the health authorities, contracts with general practitioners to provide GMS for the patients on the list of the practice. The terms and conditions of service are created through various statutes[b] and bodies, whose overall effect is a relatively (this may be under review) 'consumer-sensitive' and comprehensive service. General practitioners are self-employed, usually work in partnerships, and must offer total responsibility for the health needs, as described in GMS, of all the patients on their list. There are 'grey' areas in which GPs are allowed to charge for certain services, such as qualifying medical examinations for those on their list wishing to obtain a Heavy Goods Vehicle driving licence and other similar fitness certificates. Patients have a statutory right to a complaints procedure.

The above section explains why *healthcare* can be seen as a relatively standardised service, and the kind that most individuals requiring healthcare of any sort will recognise. The need to define or describe such services is obviated, as the training of a health professional means that members of the public have confidence that they know how to do their job, and why. It could be said that the training of such people is integral to the contract, as it describes or defines the contractual terms.

Furthermore, the work of the health professionals is frequently depicted in documentary reports and works of fiction. Colleges, which often have tremendous prestige, oversee the training of health professionals (e.g. physiotherapists) and continue to provide guidance

[b]The National Health Service Act 1977, The National Health Service (Scotland) Act 1978, Health Services Act 1980, Health and Social Security Act 1984, Health and Medicines Act 1988, NHS and Community Care Act 1990 and the Consolidation Act 1992.

through the professional membership system. Professional associations, which have access to government departments, advise members on typical fee rates for private patients.

Likewise, private clinics may provide a 'menu' of standardised services, usually surgical operations, and patients may take comfort from the fact that the private practitioners also practise in the NHS. The fact that such health professionals are trained and governed through statutory regulations provides purchasers with the confidence to proceed with obtaining their services. Contracts, which can amount to interviews with a consultant, discussions about various options and may include documents referring to times of service delivery and pay/fee rates, are more likely to be short rather than long. For the majority of purchasers of healthcare services, then, perceived outcomes are relatively clear.

However, the professions have come under criticism recently, and the Consumers' Association has published a report claiming that state and self-regulation have not produced the services most appropriate for consumers' needs. Powerful regulatory mechanisms seem to have arrived late in the day, especially with respect to the medical profession. The report examines the case for better and greater regulation.[2]

The need for definitions

But not everyone has such a clear idea of what constitutes social services, nor do they have any idea of what the staff in social services do. Social services departments provide a wide range of care and support for elderly people, people with physical disabilities, people with mental health problems, people with drugs- or alcohol-abuse problems, and ex-offenders, families and children in care. They are also responsible for the inspection and registration of care homes. The White Paper, *Modernising Social Services: Promoting Independence, Improving Protection, Raising Standards*, Cmd. 4169, describes the remit of social services, and comments: 'Often services are not planned and provided in a way that would best help service users... There is no definition of what carers can expect, nor any yardstick for judging how effective or successful Social Services are'.[3] The White Paper suggests that there is: 'a lack of clarity of objectives and standards'.

This lack of publicity and categories of services makes a market in social-care services difficult to translate into 'standard products or packages'. If a patient is discharged from hospital with a surgical wound, for example, the nurse who calls to check the wound dressing has a fairly clear task, and the lack of a properly dressed wound will soon become apparent.

There is now a blurring of nursing skills and tasks, so that the provision of healthcare may stop at ensuring that the wound – in our example – does not become infected and proceeds along a successful healing process. Nursing duties may have included a more holistic approach in the past, but there is now a marked shift to define more closely what is required of a trained nurse, and other tasks are 'relegated' to non-nurses. Such assistance may classified as 'social' care but, nevertheless, is probably associated with nurses and nursing in the mind of the general public.

Social care may mean undertaking various tasks to make the patient more comfortable; but these tasks, important as they are, have not been so recognisable to the buying public as a specialised service. Domestic cleaning is perhaps the most easily recognised, and 'personal care', as we now know it, is becoming more recognisable. Purchasing and marketing this type of service, the subject of this book, is a relatively novel concept in the supply of services. The government has, however, acknowledged its importance.

Best value

The present government published a White Paper in 1998, *Modern Local Government – In Touch with the People*, which set out proposals for modernising the entire structure and function of local government over the following 10 years. It emphasises the concept of partnership of local and central government, and of local government and its constituents, including ordinary people, local businesses and NHS organisations. It endorses ethical codes of conduct for councillors, greater involvement with people in council decisions and greater accountability, envisaging an end to compulsory competitive tendering.

This improved accountability should be transparent when local authorities make purchasing decisions, which they are exhorted to undertake with the objective of obtaining 'best value'. This 'guided' purchasing power will undoubtedly affect social services with respect to obtaining domiciliary care.

References

1 Stone J and Matthews J (1996) *Complementary Medicine and the Law.* Oxford University Press, Oxford.

2 Consumers' Association (1998) *Policy Report: Leave it to the Professionals? Professional Regulation in the 21st Century.* Consumers' Association, London.

3 Department of Health (1998) *Modernising Social Services: Promoting Independence, Improving Protection, Raising Standards,* Cmd. 4169, section 1.4. HMSO, London.

2
A general background

The government of the early 1980s had planned to improve the provision of health and social care by creating market mechanisms to increase the amount of choice to recipients of care. The NHS was restructured to form an internal market and community care was the model for social services.

Service users were to be given choices – one such choice was to have community care or care within one's own home. Residential care for elderly and disabled people was not to be the first choice of social services when it was apparent that the service user required assistance or support. Making the best of market principles, such care at home could be provided through a variety of organisations, including private sector home-care providers.

About 12 years ago, providing a 'home-care' service was a relatively little known 'cottage industry'. It was undertaken mostly by a specialised department of SSDs, and a few private and charitable suppliers took on the role of providing more specialised services, usually those not provided by the local SSD.

While the NHS and Community Care Act 1990 was in its consultation stages, it was recognised that many more organisations could supply home care, and that the set-up costs for an individual were comparatively low. Some residential and nursing homes developed a home-care service, but this was not the generality. Most new businesses require a significantly large sum of start-up capital, but providing home care required very little in the way of elaborate premises or equipment.

As the implications of the Act became more widespread, the number of small organisations providing private home care grew. The costings and profit margins of the service meant that the number of administrative staff was extremely low, and the work very demanding. As the market expanded and became more 'mature', some small organisations grew by branching out or merging with other organisations.

The various types of domiciliary (home) care on the market

There are currently a number of care providers on the market, some of which are national or regional organisations, associated with healthcare products or services. Some nursing and residential homes operate an 'outreach' service, where clients are provided with a domiciliary or home-care service and the organisation for both types of work is conducted from the nursing/residential home premises.

It is surprising that the geographical limitations of this type of care provision, and the possible benefits of localised networked services, have not led to the formation of SSD/NHS consortia, whose knowledge of the locality and local demands must be unrivalled.

However, as this type of care provision requires relatively small amounts of start-up capital, many providers operate from modest premises. Private or for-profit domiciliary care is more often provided by a care agency or a nursing agency, described in detail in Chapter 3. If specific nursing care is not required, then care workers may be divided into two categories – typically 'domestic' workers and 'personal carers'. The former will do routine cleaning, cooking, washing and so on. This is not dissimilar to the kind of work done in catering, laundry and cleaning departments within hotels, hospitals and nursing homes. 'Personal care' involves assisting an individual – known as the client or service user – in washing, dressing, bathing, feeding, etc. This type of work is not dissimilar to that undertaken by 'nursing auxiliaries' (NAs) in hospitals and nursing homes, or those at the lower levels of the trainee nurse grades.

No central register

When a nurse qualifies, she or he must apply to the United Kingdom Central Council for Nurses and Midwives (UKCC) to become a registered nurse. A record is set up – which is updated every 3 years. The qualifications, address, type and place of work are logged, and a personal identification number (PIN) is issued. An employer will seek out references as well as the PIN to check on the qualifications. But such a register is not available for workers who perform the basic caring tasks, nor does any central organisation maintain a register of organisations who provide care.

Furthermore, the Royal College of Nursing (RCN) is a professional association which provides guidance literature on numerous aspects of nursing work and lobbies the government on behalf of the nursing profession. Other trade unions, such as UNISON, undertake similar communications with government and will include non-nursing staff.

How to find out the suppliers of care

Many district nurses and GP surgeries are asked about the availability of domiciliary care, because of the lack of an accessible register. However, any information can be regarded as a recommendation and so professional people will tend to avoid naming particular organisations. GP surgeries have been asked to provide display boards for the purpose of informing patients; this is only permitted on the basis that GPs do not have a financial interest in any of the services being advertised and that the advertisements do not equate with recommendations. Many individuals must resort to the telephone book or ask their local SSD.

Large numbers of domiciliary-care providers will provide home-care services for SSDs, and the SSD staff may be able to recommend an organisation. However, as such a recommendation will allow an individual to rely on this, it is unlikely that any recommendations will be made.

Suppliers in the state system

Various local authorities across the country will have their own policies about how such domiciliary or home care is provided. Some are opposed to the idea of purchasing care from external suppliers and provide all the domiciliary or home care for their own population with SSD staff, and their priority will be to fulfil their statutory obligations to clients who have been assessed as 'in need', under section 47 of the 1990 Act.

Where possible, such SSDs may supply citizens with care on a fee-payment basis. Social services are means tested, and this is a distinguishing factor from the health services provided by the NHS. Where the client qualifies under an assessment, but his or her income and capital exceed the threshold limits, the fee chargeable for such services depends entirely on the policy of the local authority, and it is not uncommon that clients are charged a nominal fee, which does not reflect the true cost of the service. SSDs generally publish these policies, and leaflets for the public are supplied to local offices.

Where clients are offered SSD domiciliary services, otherwise known as home care, providing the choice that clients wish can be a challenging task for the organisers faced with large numbers of clients who tend to want services at the same time of the day. The organisers of the delivery of home care are likely to be a specialised level of local authority staff, often known as care managers, who need not be social workers or nurses, but whose competence extends to ensuring the adequate supply and training of the home-care workers.

The private system

Organisations providing domiciliary services such as house cleaning and laundry have been around for many years, mainly for the well heeled. They have not been prolific and not noticeably cheap. But since the inception of the 1990 Act, SSDs have a duty to stimulate positively the market in independent suppliers of care. Section 46(2)(d) of the 1990 Act requires local authorities to publish plans and consult a number of relevant organisations, including private carers, who provide care for those who qualify for SSD care provision.

The private (i.e. for profit) sector has grown considerably in the past 5 years. The organisations were more likely to have been small businesses, often run by a single person who had some previous experience of such work in the public sector. Such owners would have devoted considerable time and energy to the business.

Recently, larger organisations, not dissimilar to the high street chain shops in their organisational structure, have made more of a presence in this service. Some will be companies already established in private healthcare, owning hospitals and nursing homes.

Many of the smaller businesses have sold up to the larger organisations, with a number of consequences for the type of service. Nursing and residential homes are tending to follow the same pattern.

Charities and the not-for-profit suppliers

A number of charities have entered into the 'business' of care provision and some provide the service free of charge. They rely heavily on voluntary help, often run by people who are closely connected with the charitable cause. SSDs have 'traded' with such organisations for many years, using their services for SSD service users. Some have been in receipt of central or local government grants – and have flourished in an environment of co-operation and goodwill in the past.

But local authorities have required that they behave much more like businesses, submitting accounts and business plans. Not all the voluntary sector has approved of this bias to 'contractorisation'. The National Council for Voluntary Organisations (NCVO) has been collecting information on how SSDs have been contracting with their member organisations. They have produced a guide to contracts, *Mutual Obligations – NCVOs Guide to Contracts with Public Bodies* by Joss Saunders, Partner in Linnells Solicitors. The guide provides specific advice on dealing with contractual terms and conditions and is to be recommended to anyone who experiences difficulty in understanding a SSD contract.

Suppliers to local authority social services departments

For many private (i.e. profit-making) domiciliary-care providers, providing care services to SSDs is a large source of steady income. Such services are often purchased as a block. This is not an 'internal market' as described in Chapter 1, as it consists of an authority purchasing from the private sector, much as they might purchase street cleaning or catering.

Many services are measured in time, and buying a quantity of care hours is typically the method used here. Thus, where a SSD contracts to purchase a block of hours in a given period of time – often averaged per week and negotiated at a considerable discount – the domiciliary-care providers are then in a position to sell more care hours to the clients to whom they have already been commissioned, as well as to non-SSD clients.

The local authorities commonly use a tendering system, inviting domiciliary-care providers to send in bids to provide a specified number of care hours in a particular geographical location. Each domiciliary-care provider must make a calculation of the future costs of such an undertaking and have the certain knowledge that the requisite staff will be available for the times required. This calculation may be translated into an offer of a fixed price for a given number of hours.

An alternative system is spot purchasing, where a social worker or team leader will purchase a few care hours for a specific client. In such cases, there is often a 'global' contract between the local authority and such home-care providers, which specifies that a particular home-care provider is eligible to sell home care to the SSD, which can be commissioned by individual social workers or care managers, on the basis that various accreditation criteria have been met. This is not such a reliable source of income, although the price is not as low as it might be in the case of a block contract.

Such activity is not usually governed by the Supply of Goods and Services Act 1982 Part II, as one might expect, and which would apply to the gamut of services from installation of central heating to accountancy services. Because of the commercial risks of this type of legal relationship, this so-called 'service' is, in effect, the hiring of individuals through an agency, and the quality of service element is extremely difficult to quantify or evaluate. This topic is further discussed in Chapters 4 and 5.

Significance of SSD accreditation

It is common for SSDs to seek to accredit domiciliary-care providers in some way, before using them in either block purchasing or spot purchasing. There may be quality control checks but, more likely, accreditation will consist mainly of the successful completion of a proforma checklist or questionnaire relating to the organisational aspects, which are explained in Chapter 5, and interviews of a representative. Providers who are either accredited or publish the fact that they supply SSDs consider this to be a mark of reputability.

The interview might be for the purpose of ensuring that the private provider representative is a 'fit person'. Some SSDs will provide inspections of the offices of domiciliary-care providers and will seek to ensure the security of client information. However, that generally occurs after accreditation. They may simply use suppliers who have tendered for specific contracts.

The fine details of the service are contained within what are generally known as 'service specifications' and these may provide that any undertaking to visit a client *must* be fulfilled. But supplying more than one authority may mean that a domiciliary-care provider has to operate with two or more sets of contractual specifications, as it is unlikely that authorities will use the same purchasing criteria.

The degree of involvement by local authorities' purchasing or contracts departments will vary and SSDs will not generally be involved in the purchasing decisions if the contracts are placed through tendering. Furthermore, the procedures involved in the acceptance of tenders will not generally involve SSD staff. Procedures with respect to accepting tenders are commercially sensitive, and staff who would have a potential interest in the service are generally excluded from these deliberations. Much will depend on the way the criteria are written, and any monitoring and enforcement protocols used by the local authority SSD.

Significance of UKHCA membership

The United Kingdom Homecare Association Ltd, headquartered in Surrey, is a grant-aided (Department of Health) organisation. Through membership subscription and surveys, it represents the views of member organisations providing home care. Among its many objectives are to keep its members informed of current developments, to promote good practice and to provide technical assistance when required. It lobbies the government on issues of concern to home-care organisations and has campaigned for regulation of domiciliary-care services. It does not have a policing role and membership of the UKHCA is not evidence of conforming to any specific standards. However, member organisations, who subscribe and display their membership of the UKHCA on their brochures, are in receipt of the relevant information.

The Commission for Care Standards

The 1998 White Paper, *Modernising Social Services*, proposes the creation of Regional Committees for Care Standards, which will be independent statutory bodies. Their purpose will be to have responsibility for the regulation of a range of social services, including domiciliary social-care providers.[1] The regions will have their own inspectors, who will have skills and qualifications from both social care and healthcare. It is anticipated that there will be a constructive liaison with other regulatory agencies, such as the Health and Safety Executive, fire authorities and environmental health departments. Registration with the Commissions for Care Standards will not be mandatory, but SSDs will not place contracts with unregistered providers.

Reference

1 Department of Health (1998) *Modernising Social Services: Promoting Independence, Improving Protection, Raising Standards*, Cmd. 4169, paras 4.11–4.13. The Stationery Office, London.

3
How the suppliers are organised

The 1989 White Paper encouraged a multiplicity of suppliers of home care:

> The Government believes that the wider use of service specification and tendering is likely to be one of the most effective ways of stimulating the non-statutory sector. It has decided against extending compulsory competitive tendering to social care services, and favours giving local authorities an opportunity to make greater use of service specifications, agency agreements and contracts in an evolutionary way. The government believes that this will have the beneficial effect of requiring authorities to define desired outcomes: to be more specific about the nature of the service they are seeking to provide to achieve those outcomes; and to define the necessary inputs.[1]

As was said earlier, starting a business supplying home care has very low start-up costs compared to other related services such as nursing and residential homes, which not only involve immense capital investment in premises, but also adherence to regulatory statutes – the Registered Homes Act 1984 – and relevant regulations – The Residential Care Homes Regulations SI 1984/1345.

Furthermore, the recent trends indicate that people who are given a choice prefer to stay in their own homes until they become too disabled to cope with their own demands, rather than move to a residential home (and must also mean that those who are entering care homes are probably very frail and/or ill). Thus, as a business decision, providing home care is a growing market.

Suppliers of home care may be public limited companies, but are more likely to be private limited companies or sole traders. This means that they can trade, and enter into contracts of supply, and buy for their own businesses on negotiated terms. Thus, providers of home-care workers who wear uniforms will be able to buy uniforms from trade suppliers on special terms of business, as would any other organisation.

However, the service that they supply, that is to say care workers, can be via a number of mechanisms. The vast majority of home-care providers are agencies, governed by the Employment Agencies Act (EAA) 1973. Commercial agency is a service commonly found in selling houses and land (estate agency) and travel, but in commercial transactions is extremely common.[2] It will not always be evident to an outsider whether or not a commercial enterprise is an agency. The Department of Trade and Industry is expected to overhaul this piece of legislation for this reason.

There has often been a confusion about the person that the agency is acting for. The general high-street estate agency is usually acting for the seller, but a potential buyer may ask an estate agent to act for them in finding a suitable property. Travel agents are generally held to be acting for the consumer, while the service is being chosen, then for the tour operator after the choice has been made.[3]

Under the 1973 Act, organisations can offer workers to other organisations, either on a temporary or permanent basis. Many offices will resort to such agencies to obtain a 'temp'. An unexpected or short-term need for secretarial work is one of the most common commercial demands, and using a secretarial agency is by far the most common solution. Such agencies will often specialise in types of work, and nursing agencies, governed by the Nursing Agencies Act 1953 (and the Nurses (Scotland) Act 1951) are, in 1999, an extremely profitable enterprise.

There are a number of permutations in this triangular relationship.

- **Scenario 1**: The agency will be acting for the nurse, who is **employed** by the agency, with a contract to work a specified number of hours. The client is the organisation (e.g. a hospital) or individual who wants the nurse to do a specified job or a shift. This is generally called a principal organisation. The contract between the nurse and agency may contain a restriction such as that the nurse must not accept permanent employment from the client. The client pays the agency the requisite fee and the agency pays the nurse. This has been mirrored by some home-care agencies.

- **Scenario 2**: The agency will be acting for the nurse, who is **self-employed**, with a contract to work an unspecified number of hours. The client is the organisation (e.g. a hospital) or individual who wants the nurse to do a specified job or a shift. This is generally called an agency. The contract between the nurse and agency cannot contain a restriction such as that the nurse must not accept permanent employment from the client. The client pays the agency the requisite fee and the agency pays the nurse. This has been mirrored by most home-care agencies.

- **Scenario 3**: The agency will be acting for the nurse, who will be **employed**, with a contract to work a specified number of hours. The client is the employer (e.g. a hospital) or individual who wants the nurse to do a specified job or a shift, who will become the nurse's employer. This is generally called an agency. The contract between the nurse and agency relates to the commission charged for the introduction and placement. The employer pays the agency the requisite fee and employs the nurse. The agency drops out of the picture. This has been mirrored by some home-care agencies.

The relationship between the agency and client, be it an individual or a SSD, is governed by contract law, and is discussed in detail in Chapter 5.

The client may be an individual, such as a person who has been discharged from hospital and wants help in the home. A typical example is assistance in rising in the morning and going to bed at night. An agency that is contacted may agree to send a care worker to the client's home. The home-care worker might be a self-employed person, who obtains the client through the agency, or becomes the short-term temporary employee of the client. The details of the particular relationship should be written in the brochure of the agency organisation.

General structure of suppliers – national and local

The majority of home-care providers who started business about the time the 1989 White Paper was published, prior to the 1990 Act coming into force, were relatively small organisations with few capital assets. They were run on, perhaps, sound knowledge of the care business and considerable amounts of goodwill between the office staff and the home-care workers. As it became more evident that this was an area capable of immense expansion in business terms, some small, successful organisations started to grow, by increasing the area for which they were providing services, merging with others and spreading into newer neighbouring areas. The national charities set up branch offices in the main cities many years ago, and the care agencies that opted to grow in this way followed suit. But having a nationally or regionally known name has not always assisted in developing a service which is, of necessity, a highly localised activity.

Organisations that established a reputation in large cities took on neighbouring concerns or created franchise operations. This meant that the original staff might stay with the newly 'bought out' organisation, retaining the goodwill acquired, while reducing the risks and burdens associated with small enterprises.

The essential feature of the starter business was its name, as the goodwill associated with a name can be the most profitable asset. Thus, where a national organisation buys an existing organisation, that fact may not be made widely known to the client group. The clients of a firm generally would rely on the fact that they knew the staff well. Thus, a well-known name, associated with good care workers is a valuable asset, irrespective of a high market profile of a national organisation. There are some national organisations, within healthcare market sectors, that have instituted branches around the country.

Location of office

A supplier of home-care or nursing services does not have to be in any specific location, as the majority of business is conducted on the telephone. But the physical requirements of document storage and interviewing facilities usually mean that an office will be provided for a large city, with satellite or mini-offices servicing distant but connected areas. Small organisations may have only a single office. A large, national organisation may have a main office, which will deal with all bookkeeping and accounts, but the details of clients and matching them to home-care workers are generally kept at local level. These economies of scale should alleviate some of the administrative burdens on the local office staff.

Skills of office staff

Operating an agency is a business with a short turn-around time. That is, the transactions are based on high-volume, low-cost operations. Profitability derives from successful placements with as little 'administrative servicing' as possible once the contract has been agreed. The prime objectives at these local offices consist of finding clients and home-care workers, and servicing the former with the latter, often with very short notice. Where the main clients are SSDs, communicating with SSD staff will be an important aspect of the work. Traditionally, the staff in such offices have been nurses, but that is becoming less common. It is very important that the office staff understand the obligations under the Employment Agencies Act 1973 and the Conduct of Employment Agencies and Employment Business Regulations 1976, and the consequences of the agent–principal relationship for the staff and the client. There is no statutory requirement to have any specific qualifications, but the need to maintain a good relationship with SSD staff means that they are likely to have had nursing or social services experience.

In the large chain organisations, local staff are likely to have very little autonomy over the levels of fees charged or pay rate for the home-care workers. The centralisation of those decisions, the printing of the brochures, the raising of invoices and the computation of timesheets will mean that the office is staffed only with people concerned directly with home-care workers and clients. The profitability of the service means that there are usually very few staff who are not home-care workers. As computerised office systems become more commonly used, the office staff are also likely to have increased skills.

Relationship between office and care staff

One of the preoccupations of the office staff is to recruit home-care workers, providing appropriate induction and training and work equipment. Agencies are obliged under the 1973 Act and its regulations to ensure that the workers who are sent to clients are suitable. A well-run office will have staff who deal with recruitment and training of care workers, and another section that deals with client enquiries. Ideally, requests from the latter will be put to the former for matching. Permanent office staff will know the care workers, their availability for work, their location and their competence.

Thus, having total confidence in the training programme is essential, and the process of training often builds the relationship between the office staff and the care workers. The office is the point of contact for all 'customers', i.e. the home-care workers, the clients, SSD staff and senior personnel from the care organisation. This is the point from which enquirers should be able to obtain all the relevant information with respect to service and costs.

Organising appropriate induction and training requires sufficient time and skill, and will also depend on whether or not potential home-care workers consider it worthwhile. This is the essence of the debate on home-care provision. The demand for the service generally outstrips the supply, and finding home-care workers to service clients at their home location can be extremely problematic.

Ideally, the home-care worker who is available will live near the client, but this will rarely be the case. Home-care workers who want to work during the specific hours required by clients are few, and clients are scattered. The matching of clients to willing home-care workers consumes most of the working day in the office, and the time taken travelling between clients is usually an expense borne by the home-care worker.

Frequently, a client will ask that only one person attends them, and the provider will do what it can, but cannot offer any guarantees. The shortage of home-care workers means that there is, in reality, very little choice. The provisions in the White Paper, *Caring for People*, envisages a competitive market in this sector, with the ability to provide considerable choice to the client group, but research has shown that the service is not as widespread or sensitive to choice as envisaged.

This is due to the fluid nature of the relationships with home-care workers, who are not usually employees, are not guaranteed a weekly income and prefer to work during the hours available with respect to other commitments, such as childcare. The work offers few career development prospects and tends to be viewed as paid occupation that might fit into the life of someone who has put her or his career aside for a period.

The fact that travelling incurs quite significant expenses for a short period of working (a client may only want to have someone to attend them for 1 hour or less) leads to difficulties in the matching of home-care worker to client.

Reliance on SSD contracts

Where a home-care provider has won a contract to supply a SSD in a block contract, this can bring about some stability in the levels of work and income for the home-care workers and so such contracts are highly valued. It is important to note that in such cases, the client is the SSD and not the recipient of care services. In some organisations, home-care workers doing such work are paid at a different rate (usually lower) to private clients, but the advantage is that there is usually a large amount of SSD work compared with the private client work, and the size of the SSD block contracts, usually measured in hours, gives the local authorities tremendous bargaining power. SSDs will often negotiate a different relationship as well as lower rates, generally insisting that during the hours being worked, the home-care workers are the employees of the agency and not of the local authority. This monopolistic power to create huge demand for a service, as well as to set the charges that home-care providers can levy, is a cause of complaint.[4] The reasons for this will be explained in Chapters 5 and 6.

Relationship between office and others, such as health professionals

Home-care workers do not generally work in isolation in an individual's house. The client is likely to be under the supervision of the SSD or the district nurse, or in a warden-controlled flat in a sheltered housing unit. Calling on such a person at regular intervals will inevitably lead to communication with the others who also do similar things (known as care staff or having similar descriptions). It is eminently sensible that all such care staff co-operate, and this relationship is invariably a positive one.

However, these communications do not arise spontaneously out of a 'common-sense' desire to act in the interests of the clients. The client is usually under the supervening authority who is responsible for this aspect of necessary co-ordination, i.e. the SSD. Unless the client has chosen to organise his or her own home-care worker, a social worker will be able to direct or maintain vigilance on the many callers to a client's home.

When this vigilance fails, then the inevitable problems, such as calling at the wrong time, will occur. Thus, not only are there geographical problems, related to where the client and home-care worker live, but also problems related to correct timing. Where nurses and other health professionals visit the client, usually to perform specific tasks, it may be that the presence of the home-care worker is an advantage. The home-care worker may be asked to assist the former and information about the client may be voiced. A NHS nurse or physiotherapist will have no authority to request a home-care worker to do specific tasks unless specified in the contract for care, and the home-care worker may be placed in an invidious situation.

The question of 'liaison' and client confidentiality

Disclosures about the clients, either from the clients themselves or from care staff, can be extremely problematic. Inevitably, staff will need to know a few intimate details if personal care is being provided, but do unconnected staff have a right to discuss such matters amongst themselves? This is often a cause of complaint from clients. Most home-care workers will not have a thorough training in maintaining client confidentiality.

The relationship between the client and home-care worker is a contractual one, and the ethical implications of maintaining client confidentiality have not been fully addressed, either by SSDs or by the Department of Health. Nurses attending a patient who is also in receipt of home care do not have any obligations to divulge confidential information about the client/patient to the home-care worker and may be in breach of their code of confidentiality if they do disclose such information when the patient has not consented expressly to any such disclosure.

The home-care provider's terms and conditions of service will indicate whether or not confidentiality is an integral part of the service, but if the home-care worker is working on a self-employed basis, there are inherent difficulties in monitoring the training necessary to ensure a truly confidential service. Moreover, poorly trained workers may not accept that a client or service user has a right to keep confidential information, such as their HIV status.

Record keeping

Any organisation must keep records, and providing a service usually requires intensive recording of details. Where SSDs contract with home-care providers, the terms and conditions of the contract, often called the service specifications, will require stringent attention to the way records are made and stored, including their security.

If the organisation does not contract with SSDs, then the Employment Agencies Act 1973 regulations provide that detailed records are maintained. There are statutory rights for the subjects to ensure that any details kept about them on a computer are correct, and under the new Data Protection Act 1998 all files on living people will be governed by the Act. Thus all organisations providing home care are statutorily obliged to keep the client records secure and up to date.

Security for file storage is extremely important, as names and addresses of a vulnerable sector of the population are maintained, along with the reason for requiring home care, such as a particular disability, and the details relating to accessing the client's home via electronic entry codes, and so on.

Family details, such as next of kin, with their addresses, will also be on record. The appropriate use of this information is vital to the success of a good quality service. However, keeping records up to date is a time-consuming task and is often placed on the shoulders of already over-burdened office staff.

Other records that are vital to the business of home-care providers are the tally of the care-hours undertaken, so that a client can be invoiced and the careworker paid. The majority of care workers are paid for the work that they have done, and the records for this are central to the business, as evidence of the transactions. These transactions are generally computed in hours, which must be logged at least three times – against the client, against the care worker and for the business accounts. Moreover, the clients may have purchased differently priced packages and the careworker may have worked for a variety of pay rates. Again, this highly time-consuming task has to be undertaken by office staff, and where the larger organisations have a central processing office, this activity is usually undertaken centrally.

Such levels of automation can mean great difficulties in addressing problems related to accounting errors. Errors will tend to occur when changes and cancellations are badly processed. The business is a volume-based enterprise and, therefore, only profitable on the basis of large numbers of hours being 'sold' successfully. Such automated systems require a great deal of skill in resolving errors. Computations of these transactions are generally undertaken by staff using accounts software, and so errors made before the inputting of data has begun are difficult to trace and correct.

Ideally, clients should be billed on a regular basis, with a prior agreement to pay at specified intervals. There are inevitable circumstances where a client continues to request home care without actually paying his or her bills. This should not affect payment of the home-care worker. When a client dies in debt to the home-care agency, the agency generally will pursue the executors or personal representatives for the amount outstanding.

Confidentiality

This has been one of the greatest areas of complaint and poor management. The geographical problems related to a domiciliary service are often the unwillingness of home-care workers to travel any great distance and, for economic reasons, it is preferable for them to see several clients inhabiting the same locality, in which the home-care worker may also live.

Communications between client and care worker should be kept confidential between them, and if a matter of concern is raised, the care worker will be advised to follow a proper procedure.

Details of one client should never be communicated to another. Where clients of a single home-care provider do live in proximity to each other, breaches of communication can not only lead to embarrassment, but to poor security. This problem can only be addressed through proper training and the adoption of ethical principles.

Level of skill of care workers

Care workers are a scarce resource, and a recently published figure indicated a national shortage of 8000 people in the healthcare services alone. The scarcity in social care work is even more severe, and in the business of home-care providers is exacerbated by the need for mobility.

The work is low paid and irregular, workers generally only get paid for what they do, and maintaining their own private transport is an enormous expense. This work must be seen in the light of the possibility of doing regular shifts in a nursing home or hospital. The requirement for fairly intense levels of training, during which the pay might be less than normal hourly pay, is a challenge for most home-care providers. Furthermore, the average period of time that a care worker will remain with a home-care provider is very short, perhaps a few months.

Care workers who are untrained are a risk to themselves as well as to the clients they attend. Most home-care providers will insist that care workers undergo training in manual handling, as transferring clients from place to place within the home is a common aspect of the service.

Surveys on the skill levels of such care workers are difficult, but where documentary evidence has been produced, the home-care providers in the independent sector are shown to lag behind the SSD staff and those in the not-for-profit organisations.

Training in basic social care can lead to the award of a National Vocational Qualification (NVQ) level 2. After a period of training, a trained assessor observes that the candidate can perform a given list of tasks. These include enabling the client to maintain personal cleanliness, enabling clients to eat and drink, and assisting in minimising client discomfort and pain. This is not an exhaustive list. However, lack of financial incentives for trained care workers will affect their willingness to undertake the training. But more likely, the irregularity of the work will determine a worker's willingness to work with a particular home-care provider.

Paying for a qualified person to assess other staff for their competence will be another significant expense for a firm providing care. Only those firms dedicated to providing a quality service, and who may charge more than the lowest prices, will be in a position to assess their care staff.

Nursing qualifications

Frequently a home-care provider will seek to maintain standards by employing a qualified nurse as a senior person in the organisation. Nurses who maintain their UKCC registration, evidenced by a pin number and the letters 'RGN' or 'RMN', will have sound knowledge of training requirements and will probably be involved in training care workers. A qualified nurse, implementing the UKCC code of ethics, provides clients with some confidence that quality standards will be upheld.

However, nursing in a hospital or nursing home is not necessarily similar to caring for a client in his or her own home. The purpose of the domiciliary care is not necessarily cure – rather, the goals can be much more diffuse. Home care is usually required by patients to help them live the life they wish to lead, in spite of any illness, disability or difficulties. The training that nurses undergo will have a different set of priorities, and is often specialty based (theatre nurses, for example). But it is important that there is a professionally qualified person within the organisation who will understand the level of risks and the need for appropriate training.

Regulation in the future

No statute is in force to ensure the quality of the people who provide home care. This omission has been raised in Parliament, and the Registration of Domiciliary Care Agencies Bill 1993 was given a first reading in the House of Commons, but failed to make it to the statute books. More recent government ministers in the Department of Health confirmed their intention to regulate this sector, and the present Secretary of State for Heath, Mr Frank Dobson, has published a White Paper, *Modernising Social Services*, which includes a promise to introduce a regulatory system for domiciliary care as described in previous chapters.

When a client comes to depend on a care worker coming to his or her home and providing much-needed assistance or relief, the relationship can be more disempowering than empowering, in spite of the fact that the relationship between the client and the paid carer is often, but not always, an unequal one. Typical unequal professional relationships are doctor/patient, nurse/patient, solicitor/client, etc., and a code of ethics is implanted in the training of such professional people, invariably enforced through statutory obligations. Thus, reported breaches are dealt with by a formal disciplinary system. Social services staff appear as the exception to this general concept of ethical codes of professional conduct, an issue that has been examined in a report *Safe-guarding Standards* by Professor Roy Parker (1990). The White Paper *Modernising Social Services* proposes a new statutory body – the General Social Care Council (GSCC) – which will approximately mirror the UKCC for nurses and will: 'set conduct and practice standards for all social services staff, and register those in the most sensitive areas … The constitution of the GSCC, its methods of operation and the arrangements for its governance will reflect a paramount general duty to serve the interests and the welfare of service users and the confidence of the public'.[5]

References

1 Department of Health and Social Services (1989) *Caring for People: Community Care in the Next Decade and Beyond*, Cmd. 849, para. 3.4.7. HMSO, London.

2 Bradgate R (1995) *Commercial Law*. Butterworths, London.

3 Grant D and Mason S (1995) *Holiday Law*. Sweet and Maxwell, London.

4 Department of Health (1993) *Monitoring and Development – A Special Study of Purchasing and Contracting*. HMSO, London.

5 Department of Health (1998) *Modernising Social Services*, Cmd. 4169. The Stationery Office, London.

4
Choosing a supplier of care: price

The pricing of any service takes into account the wages due to the worker providing the service, any materials supplied with the service and the market's capacity to pay a certain price. The first of these – wages – will also be related directly to the scarcity of that particular type of worker.

An example is a computer software designer who knows how to write a program that meets the needs of an organisation. As these types of worker are rare, and the demand for them is high, they will be inclined to demand high wages, or large fees; large organisations will be prepared to pay the increased cost, as the economic pressure to obtain their services outweighs the cost of the service.

Nurses can command relatively high wages outside the NHS, working for agencies or private homes. Nursing agencies currently contract with the NHS, which, for numerous reasons related to absenteeism, planning and resources, 'buys' in agency nurses. The NHS pays these agency nurses a considerably higher hourly rate than it pays its own staff. Few private individuals are prepared to pay for a nurse at the agency rates, which can be over £9.00 per hour.

Care staff are usually paid considerably less than nurses, and the shortage of such staff does not appear to affect their wages in the same way as described for software designers. The ability or inability to pay the high wages is the restricting market force. In the present system, the buyers are mainly SSDs or individuals, and the former have well-publicised resource limitations.

The latter, the private client, will have a wide spectrum of ability to pay. There are the well heeled, who perhaps have always paid for help in the home, and for whom pricing is not the main criterion. There is the middle range of working people, who perhaps need some help at a particular point because of illness or disability – often of a temporary nature. They will tend to buy according to price. But by far the largest sector of buyers comprises elderly people, often with a specific disability, such as arthritis, whose income is below the national average.

Pricing structure

Such individuals will often be SSD clients, and SSD care services are available only on the basis of means testing. It is this sector, along with SSDs themselves, that tends to dictate the pricing structure. In order to tender for a SSD contract, home-care providers must prepare a competitive bid, which, if accepted, means that the organisation is held down to a fairly low price, where the profit margin is extremely narrow.

The price of the service, expressed as an hourly rate, pays for the wages of the care workers, plus the agency commission. The services are currently divided into 'packages', such as:

- domestic, includes cleaning, laundry, cooking

- personal care, includes assisting with bathing, dressing, etc.

- sleeping-in, where a care worker is expected to sleep most of the night, but must be prepared to be woken and provide personal care

- night attendance, where a care worker would be expected to remain awake and attend for most of the night

- live-in care worker.

The first two 'packages' tend to be priced by the hour and, often, the way SSDs are prepared to pay determines the package structures provided by the private care agencies. More imaginative care packages could be available, and would depend on the care agency having the freedom and individuality to create them.

The commission must pay for overheads of administration, after which sufficient profits must be realised to make the enterprise worthwhile. Where a large organisation has local branches, these overheads are minimised by centralised administrative services, as described in Chapter 2. Nevertheless, the hourly rate paid by a client must cover the whole of the staff salary bill, plus the costs of premises, services and working materials. Telephone bills are a large component of the non-wage costs.

Firms that wish to have the stability provided by a large SSD contract will attempt to offer the lowest possible price, which in retrospect might seem unrealistic, especially in the light of any other quality standards that might also be imposed, such as a guarantee of the service. Such a guarantee may mean that the organisation can never make cancellations. Given that staff shortages are an occupational hazard, this is a high-risk undertaking. An often-used penalty is termination of the contract. But without a large SSD contract that keeps the care workers in work, an organisation is unlikely to have enough care workers for any clients at all. SSDs can be reluctant to commit themselves to buying into the future, for unallocated care services. A contract between SSD and supplier for a long-term 'block' can act as a restriction in client choice. There is unlikely to be a comparable large, regular, private demand for home care.

However, growth of the private long-term care insurance market could lead to significant changes in provision of home care. Although, currently, pricing in the private sector may be a market variable, in reality the private sector is not large enough to sustain anything other than fairly small organisations, which will often pride themselves on good local knowledge and access to reliable care workers. Those who have built up reputations with a private client sector, and whose prices reflect that market, are not usually prepared to accept SSD contracts. Equally, their care workers may only take on clients who are from the private sector.

The range of prices reflects the range of services – from cleaning only, to more complex social services such as companionship, personal services in bathing and dressing, or assisting with wound or catheter care. A significant sector of the market wants a sleep-in service, which means that a care worker is required to stay overnight and assist in case the client wakes. This is most commonly requested when the family member(s) who provides the care during the day wants to ensure a night's rest. Some organisations also provide a live-in service, which can be for a companion to stay with someone for the most of the week, or someone who takes on quite specific duties related to the client's personal needs, such as continence and mobility assistance.

Connection of carer pay to price of service

There is a close connection between the price charged and the care worker's wages. The price of the packages determines the care worker's pay level, and so doing domestic work, the cheapest package, will yield the lowest rate for the care worker. But the difference in hourly pay rates is not very significant. The generality is that the care worker is self-employed, and the total fee charged will be the combination of the carer's pay, plus travelling expenses, plus the commission due to the agency for the service of introducing a care worker. This introductory service fee will include the costs of training the care workers.

Some SSD contracts require a large number of clients to be serviced in a particular aspect. Examples are assisting clients to get out of bed or into bed, and, on the basis that these services need not take a long time, SSDs want to pay only for the time taken to do the task. Thus, a SSD contract might require a service for less than 1 hour – perhaps even half or a quarter of an hour. Many home-care providers advertise that they will provide this 'unit' of care service, but it may be unrealistic from the point of view of the care worker, especially where travel time and costs are involved.

However, where a care worker is required for a long period, such as 4 or more hours, this can be advantageous to a care worker, and so such a contract might be easier to fulfil. SSDs are generally aware that home-care providers can ill afford to sustain contracts for very small units of service.

Discounting

Any client, whether an individual or a SSD, can attempt to negotiate a discount for a bulk purchase, as regular work is highly valued. It helps in stabilising the availability of the care workers. When SSDs make a block purchase, it is at a discount (i.e. the price per hour is less than the advertised price). Having a 24-hour, live-in service is often negotiated at a discount.

SSDs generally buy at a lower price than an individual client, and this offer to buy at a fixed price is the key factor in the near monopolistic powers of SSDs. Such prices are fixed at an annual rate review, often dictated by the SSD. SSDs will set their budgets for purchasing care in the light of their present expenditure and estimated future expenditure. They must make provision for large numbers of their population who, under means testing, will become eligible for care services.

Private individuals will usually be charged a higher advertised rate, which will reflect the actual cost of the service more accurately.

Description of service

The word 'care' is not defined in the 1990 Act in isolation. In section 46(3) there is reference to 'community care services', which are those services that a local authority may provide under any of the following provisions: Part III of the National Assistance Act 1948; section 45 of the Health Services and Public Health Act 1968; section 21 of and Schedule 8 to the National Health Service Act 1977; and section 117 of the Mental Health Act 1983.

The 1989 White Paper, paragraph 1.1, explains that community care is the provision of support for people who are affected by the problems of ageing, mental illness, mental handicap, or physical or sensory disabilities, in order for them to live as independently as possible in their own homes, or in 'homely' settings in the community. The advertising literature for private home-care providers tends to be couched in this vague language, and a more detailed description of the type of service being delivered will become apparent when setting up a care plan.

A care plan is usually a task-based list of activities, in which the details may be articulated, but not necessarily all written down. Examples of the task list are: assist with rising at a specific time; assist with toiletting or bathing; dressing; meal preparation; shopping and so forth. The care plan becomes the basis of the contractual arrangements between the agency and the client, and also between the client and the care worker. It should specify clearly, in ordinary language, who the care worker is, what the duties of the care worker will be, the dates and times of the day, how the care worker is to gain access to the client's home, the price including VAT, and any other relevant factors of the service.

Depending on the precise contractual relationship between the parties, the client is usually purchasing the services from an individual on the basis of the representations made by the agency. It is possible, but unlikely, that the care plan may be created by the care worker who will be attending. Furthermore, a representative from the agency should explain the legal relationships that will arise in the event of the contract being agreed. An agency will declare that it is only liable for the actions of persons in its direct employment in work-related activity (but *see* Chapter 5). Thus, agencies will generally not accept liability for self-employed care workers. SSDs are in a position to renegotiate this, and the service specifications usually provide that while an agency care worker is with a SSD client, known as a service-user, the care worker is in the employment of the agency and so liability cannot be avoided.

Difficulties with respect to liabilities can arise when a care worker is required for a person who is mentally ill or incompetent, and the provider organisation should understand the full nature of the client's ability to consent. Attending such clients is generally only undertaken by care workers with training and experience of working with mental illness. Purchasers of care services should be confident that any care worker who takes on such a client is properly trained.

Travelling time – punctuality

The method of obtaining domiciliary care is that the person providing the care travels to the client's home, and this can be problematic, especially when the care worker attends many clients. Sufficient time must be allowed for the care worker to arrive at the specified time in the client's home. Otherwise, the agreement between the agency and client must include a provision for the time taken in travelling.

However, where a care worker is late, there can be a consequential series of problems if any other care providers are also scheduled to call, such as district nurses or physiotherapists. It is important to include information relating to such appointments while setting up the care plan in order to alert the agency that timeliness is very important.

Such detail, although not necessary for the care worker *per se*, enables the appropriate level of priority to be attached to the appointment. For some clients, a fixed time to attend will not be important, and it is helpful while drawing up the care plan to choose a 'window' of time, e.g. any 2 hours between 1.00 p.m. and 4.00 p.m., to provide flexibility where is it is needed. With respect to cancellations, purchasers should note the notice period required. Cancelling a visit at the last minute might mean that the care worker will not be paid any expenses for a fruitless journey.

Travelling is also problematic where a client is not located near to any other client or care worker. If considerable distances are involved for a short duration, it is likely that the agency will consider serving such a client as unprofitable. Although travel expenses are paid to the care workers, they are not usually paid for the time taken in travelling.

Invoicing

The process of invoicing should be clearly explained when the care plan is being agreed, and invoices should be plainly understood. The intervals at which they are sent, together with an explanation of the charges and the time available to pay them, should be included in the care plan. It has been the case that the client cannot be invoiced until the care worker has completed the work and obtained a signed document from the client to this fact. This can lead to invoices being sent to the client later than had been envisaged in the agreement. The various rates for the different care packages and the varying rates of pay due to the care worker can add further complications. SSDs will frequently expect invoices to be sent within a specific period of time and object to late invoices.

Budgeting for such bills can be difficult for clients, but setting up standing orders or direct debits should only be undertaken with sound financial advice. They are generally more difficult to cancel if the service ceases.

Time to pay

It is useful to ask if payments can be made on specific dates, which may not correspond with invoice dates. If a client is in receipt of a grant or is a beneficiary of a trust, such payments can be periodic or quarterly, and asking for time to pay should be addressed at the time the care plan is being agreed.

Under the local authority statutory regulation, SI 734/1997, *The Community Care (Direct Payments) Regulations 1997*, which came into force on 1 April 1997, enables local authorities to make direct payments to persons eligible for community care services, in order that such persons may purchase the services themselves. However, there is a long list of exceptions to this receipt of payment, including persons aged 65 or over, unless they were in receipt of such payment in the 12 months immediately before their 65th birthday (Regulation 2(2)(a) SI No 734 1997). But recent guidance states that the government is considering including people over 65 in the Direct Payment Scheme. There may also be a possibility for 'topping up'. Although originally related to residential care, SSD current guidance is that third parties may be able to top up payments by the local authority if the preferred service is more expensive than the local authority provision.

Those in receipt of such monies are advised to consult with their local advisory groups or the organisations listed in the Appendix at the end of this book on the availability and quality of home-care providers if there are doubts about the optimum methods of obtaining home-care services.

Insurance to cover long-term care

Many types of policy provide for future care in a limited way. It is a familiar concept in dentistry, where enrolment in a scheme involves an examination by a dentist who participates in the scheme. The candidate is graded according to the state of their dental health and informed that participation in the scheme will cost a fixed amount per month for a fixed period. This is generally renewable annually, and the premium can change through inflation-indexed calculations and/or the state of dental health. The scheme offers a number of consultations per year, with a range of treatments if necessary. Treatment excluded from the scheme, e.g. cosmetic work, should be clearly specified.

However, care provided at home is not so definable a service as dentistry. Nevertheless, the insurance industry has devised a number of financial products and awaits government announcements on the future of pensions and state-funded long-term care. In a previous discussion paper, in 1996, the government at that time had invited consultation on the idea of the state forming a partnership with financial institutions to address the problem of the rising costs of long-term care for a population that was becoming increasingly elderly. The common method of enabling an indemnity insurance scheme was viewed as problematic:

> *Long term care insurance has been available in the United Kingdom since 1991, but relatively few policies have been sold. One of the obstacles in selling more is that although most people who need long term care need it for a relatively short period, some need care for many years. This makes it difficult to price policies which offer indefinite cover, which tends to make them more expensive. Policies which offer cover for only a limited period are easier to price, the consumers may find them less attractive if they think there is a risk that the insurance benefit will run out while they still need care.*[1]

In spite of the calculation of risk, the insurance industry has subsequently developed a range of products. The number of people in residential care is falling, after a peak in 1995, and this may account for a resurgence in creative thinking on the funding of care in old age. Currently there are three types of policy, but this is a fluid picture, and insurers wait to hear the new plans for state-funded care by the government.

- **Type 1**: this is a straightforward indemnification where the purchaser pays premiums or a lump sum and if long-term care is required, then the policy can be activated. Generally these premiums are not payable when a claim is in force. If no claims are made, the premiums paid out by the purchaser cannot be reclaimed. In this respect, this type of policy operates like a house buildings or house contents or car insurance. A variety of this type is a health-linked life insurance policy, which can be triggered to pay out if any of the named conditions in the list is suffered by the insured. The benefit can be spent on anything, such as mortgage repayments.

- **Type 2**: some policies, in acknowledgement of the lower risks of claims being made, provide for an investment element. This type of product has been designed specifically to fund long-term care, and if the insurer dies before the fund is exhausted the remainder is included in their estate and so can be passed on to the heirs.

- **Type 3**: policies have been devised to provide for immediate care and tend to be expensive. They involve handing over a sizeable sum of money to the insurer, who will invest it and provide the insured with sufficient income to pay for long-term care.

Pricing levels can be established by looking at the way claims are triggered. The insurance companies use a task-based list called Activities of Daily Living (ADLs). These include washing oneself, dressing oneself, feeding oneself, being able to move around in your home, toiletting and continence care. The inability to perform a number of ADLs can trigger a claim. The cheaper types of insurance will be the ones where the trigger clause involves the inability to perform several ADLs (e.g. three or more). The more expensive policies will be triggered by the inability to perform two or one ADLs. Those who intend to purchase insurance-based care plans are strongly advised to seek advice from an independent financial adviser.[2] The institution set up to regulate most financial products is the Personal Investment Authority (1 Canada Square, Canary Wharf, London E14 5AZ; Tel: 0171 538 8860). Not all companies who market long-term care products are regulated by the PIA. For those who intend to purchase care, there are a number of questions to bear in mind when investigating the value of any care policy. The questions that should be asked are:

- How can I guarantee that any of the companies selling long-term care insurance will still be in existence when I need my care?

- Will premiums stay the same?

- Who will decide what care is needed?

- What happens if there is a disagreement?

- Is a medical examination required?

- Are premiums set according to the state of health of the insured?

- How will payment be made to me in the event of a claim being triggered?

- To whom will the payments be made? (payments have tended to be made to institutions or nursing homes in the past)

- How much will the payments be – is there a maximum?
- Are they subject to abatement on the payment of any other benefits or policies?
- How many ADLs are used to trigger the claim?
- Will a care counsellor be available?
- Will the insurer set up a care plan and, if so, with whom?
- Can I spend the money on anything, e.g. holidays, physiotherapy?
- Can I pay a member of my family or anyone else to care for me?
- Can I pay for someone to give my own carer a break?

References

1 Department of Health (1996) *A New Partnership for Care in Old Age: A Consultation Paper*, Cmd. 3242. HMSO, London.

2 Cowie I (1998) *Daily Telegraph, Sunday Telegraph Guide to Long Term Care*. Free Publishing Services, London.

5
Choosing a supplier of care: quality

The aspect of quality is the most hotly debated issue, intimately connected to price, in the free market provision of home care, and it is the stated aim of the UKHCA to promote a quality service. Detecting quality can be difficult, given that the service does not need any physical manifestation.

Its nature means that it is invisible to outside eyes, unlike a nursing or residential home where a visitor can see the condition of the premises, staff and inhabitants. Recipients of home care are probably not a vocal consumer group, and the scarcity of the service means that clients are unlikely to relinquish the one that they have.

SSDs who make a 'block contract' arrangement with a private provider will often use the providers for subsequent cases on a 'spot purchase' basis. The fact that the home-care provider is already a supplier enables social workers, home-care team leaders and so forth to access the provider rapidly, but the following procedures are similar for all new service users.

When purchasing care initially, the contact will be made by a person in the office. As offices are a relatively large expense, the trend is for a single office to provide services to a wide geographical area, and so making a visit to the office may not be a practical consideration for most potential purchasers. Health- and social-care professionals who are responsible for purchasing will probably undertake all transactions over the phone and will rarely meet the representative from the home-care provider. But where an organisation has been dealt with by other departmental staff, the importance of meeting will recede slightly.

Each new client (the recipient of care) should be visited, for a number of reasons. This is the opportunity to evaluate the organisation before committing oneself to the purchase. It is suggested here that when a health- or social-care professional wishes to purchase care or assist with a purchase, a meeting is held at the home of the client or patient. This meeting provides the opportunity for a face-to-face evaluation and a chance to ask questions in an unhurried way, which can give useful clues as to the quality of the organisation. Although SSD service users are outside the contract, they should be consulted. Under the Best Value criteria recently endorsed by the government, local authorities must seek to ensure that contracts are placed with appropriate contractors on the basis that the service provided is acceptable to the actual recipients. The importance of the organisation's representative who attends this meeting cannot be underestimated, as this will probably be the only opportunity to examine the way the organisation functions.

Furthermore, it is useful to examine the paperwork, including the brochure, in order to ascertain the applicability of the written information to the present case. This is extremely useful when a tailor-made service is being considered. The representative from the organisation will indicate the strengths of that organisation and discuss how they can provide the service for the case in hand. The majority of the services fall into domestic work and personal care categories, provided for a specified number of hours per day or week.

How does the organisation establish the customer's needs?

Establishing the client's needs can be daunting for all concerned, depending on whether or not the client is paying for her or his own care. Where a statutory body is purchasing care for a client, a number of factors come into play.

Does the client want anyone to call at his or her home? The health- or social-care worker who has been assigned the case will generally have the responsibility of undertaking the 'assessment of needs', and this may not coincide with the client's own view. Once it has been established that the client does want and need someone to call, the next stage is to consider who will call to do what.

A care plan is drawn up, in consultation with the client. Ideally this should be a document with the heading 'Care plan' to distinguish it from other documents. Any family member who undertakes the role of carer should also be consulted. It has been said that this army of dedicated people – usually family members – saves the Treasury a considerable sum of money.[1] The Carers (Recognition and Services) Act 1995 provides that the needs of such carers looking after older people must also be assessed. SSDs will decide whether the client can be dealt with by SSD home-care staff or whether the home care must be purchased.

Such are the choices facing SSDs, and there is a range of policies across the country as to the type of organisation that will provide the care. Some SSDs have a policy not to purchase home care from private providers, while others have 'contracted out' the entire home-care operation. Many SSDs occupy a middle position, where the in-house staff will undertake most of the work or a significant proportion of the work, and only peripheral aspects are 'purchased' from external providers. Commonly, SSD staff will be able to provide services between 9 a.m. and 5 p.m., Monday to Friday, and where services are required out of those hours, external providers may be used. It is not uncommon for SSDs to use the combination of service providers to meet the needs of a service user for 24 hours a day, 7 days a week. Thus a service user may be 'inflicted' with visits from a range of organisations, creating the possibility of confusion. During weekends especially, where problems arise, it might be difficult to contact SSDs in order to confirm any arrangements.

While adopting the task-based approach that has been described earlier, the performance of the numerous organisations would have been measured against the criteria in the care plan, such as timeliness, courteousness, etc. The task-based approach is not necessarily an empowering concept, especially as cash-strapped SSDs contract for 10-minute visits, in which the service user is transferred, or put to bed, or assisted with toileting needs.

The voluntary sector and the not-for-profit sector are used heavily. Charities, which may have been set up as pressure groups, usually specialised in a particular aspect of disability, are not always willing to contract with SSDs. It has been said that the conditions by which the SSDs wish to conduct business are too stringent, and that the charitable purpose is deflected by the necessity to create business plans and pay a management and accountancy tier inside the organisation.

The private home-care provider, who is commissioned by a health- or social-care worker has a difficult path to tread – the health- or social-care purchaser will have decided on the limit of the budget for the case in hand. Generally, the limits of expenditure are connected to the cost of institutional care, and when the cost of home care reaches the cost of institutional care, the service user may have to decide on the latter.

The budget for home care usually buys care hours, and thus the calculation of the number of hours per client is the critical factor in making the decision. Hopefully, the client will be persuaded of that view, and where the possibility of a worsening situation arises, monies must be held back to pay for a greater number of hours in the future. The health- or social-care purchaser then, in effect, subcontracts the responsibility for providing the home care to the agency, who in turn subcontracts to a home-care worker.

It is unlikely that every client will know of this arrangement, but nevertheless, the home care must be provided according to the care plan drawn up between the purchaser, the agency and the client. The possible scenario that may follow is that the client asks the home-care worker to stay longer, do more or different tasks than were agreed in the care plan or other deviations from the plan, which invariably effect a cost to the organisation providing home care.

It must be borne in mind that the client and the organisation providing home care are not in a contractual relationship with one another and that the contract is between the purchaser and the home care-providing organisation at a pre-arranged fee rate.[a] When such deviations occur, the goodwill of the home-care worker is tested, and he or she may feel that this is not the job for him or her. This will be a particularly hazardous likelihood where the home-care worker is new or the client is overbearing. The home-care worker will not be in a position to redress such a delicate and sensitive matter until contact is made with the home-care office. The dynamic within the office is driven by the business pressure to increase turnover. The solution for the organisation is to inform the purchaser of such events and to trust that extra work will command an additional or supplementary payment. This type of event is not uncommon and causes bureaucratic delays. Existing complex billing procedures are further complicated, reinforcing the need for good, effective communication within an organisation.

Of course, the care worker may be the source of problems, by being late, leaving early or by poor workmanship, for example. The client is generally informed of complaint procedures and can complain to the private home-care provider or to the purchaser. Where the client is the purchaser, the contract can be terminated.

Where there is high staff turnover, both at administrative and operational levels, the communications gap is bound to widen. The ratio between staff and clients is relevant here, in determining the quality of the service. The drive to increase business is often transmitted through a widening of this ratio. In business jargon, this is a low-cost, high-turnover enterprise, and increasing contact time between adminis-

[a]The Common Law Rules of Privity of Contract provide that contractual rights accrue only when consideration has passed between the parties, and so beneficiaries of contractual arrangements who have not provided any consideration cannot sue upon the contract.

trators, supervisors and care managers within an organisation, and between the purchaser and provider, is not usually considered as profitable. But where SSD contracts are valued, considerable efforts are invested in building relationships with SSD staff.

How does the organisation staff the service?

An agency is on a permanent recruitment drive. Some agencies publish their membership of the Federation of Recruitment and Employment Services (FRES). The Federation offers services to its members, mainly in the form of sending lists of agencies to job seekers. This applies irrespective of the kind of service the agency ultimately provides, because that is the central nature of the business.

Agencies covered by the Employment Agencies Act 1973 are in the business of 'selling' people who are willing to work to anyone who wants them, for the purpose of specified work. The majority of home-care providers have adopted the business entity of agency, because selling a 'home-care service' has considerably more business risks attached to it, with respect to liability in health and safety, and financial stability. Buyers or purchasers of such a service will accrue considerably more legal rights in contract law. Employees of such an organisation will accrue employment rights. However, if the risk can be judged as not significant, then providing a direct service where the care workers are the permanent staff of the organisation, or are all partners, has the potential of maintaining higher standards of quality.

SSDs generally purchase from care agencies on the basis of purchasing a service, as opposed to hiring staff, and the contract is a detailed service specification. Included in the terms and conditions may be a paragraph which clearly announces that the SSD will consider the home-care provider as the principal. This reduces the tiers of subcontracting and means that the care provider organisation will be directly responsible for all the acts and omissions of its staff, including the home-care workers. Thus, a care-provider organisation cannot remain blameless for a poor service by its care workers.

The recruitment aspect of care agencies leads to the search for particular person profiles, and some are more preferable than others, based on reliability and availability. The extreme shortage in the hospital and residential/nursing home sectors will mean that available people who want to take up care as a career move are rare. Thus, the agencies have to look to sectors where people will take up employment as home-care workers if the available work fits in with their own time schedules. The vast majority are mothers and students who want part-time work and are not totally dependent on the income from that work. It is not uncommon that such part-time workers will have higher priorities than home-care work. Mothers of young children have to deal with their children being sick, and at home during school holidays. Students tend to be temporary workers, by dint of the length of the academic terms.

Another serious problem from the point of view of planning is that the staff turnover is very high. Those who need a guaranteed income will move on if the agency fails to find them regular work. The reliable staff will tend to stay with a handful of clients, even if there is some travelling, provided that they have a good relationship and as long as there is a degree of regularity in the work slots.

Thus, the agency nature of the relationship in the organisation, and poor levels of pay and of other benefits, mitigate against the ability to guarantee a care worker. In other similar organisations which send workers to private premises (e.g. for appliance repairs), the worker is likely to be a reasonably paid, skilled tradesman, who is paid a regular wage. The perception of the work to a potential workforce will determine the commitment that any care worker will have to doing a good job. The vast majority of home-care workers are very committed to the policy of providing home care and to the independence that this service brings to clients.

The administrative staff are therefore performing a constant juggling act, attempting to match up workers and clients, and to develop sound relationships with bulk SSD purchasers, who are represented by individual social workers or care managers.

How does the organisation perform the risk assessment?

Before any agreement is drawn up, a representative from the home-care agency must be able to understand and quantify the risks for both parties. The client's own health and the condition of the premises must allow for the services to be delivered. A fairly standard questionnaire is produced, and as the questioner works her or his way through the form, it gives both parties the opportunity to explore the relevant factors that pose hazards and risks. This can be a difficult situation, particularly if the client does not wish to divulge any medical history. There is no question of compulsion, and the reasoning is that care workers should be informed of the risk of such ailments (an example being a heart condition which might mean that the client is likely to have a heart attack). However, most working people who have domestic help in the house might consider it to be an infringement of their privacy to be asked questions about their health. Thus, this sensitive issue is related to the needs of the service user and is difficult to evaluate in the free-market ethos.

Where a care worker provides the client or service user with personal services of washing and bathing, the lack of mobility of the client is an essential piece of information, and diseases of the joints and muscles that give rise to the immobility must be documented and understood in order that the personal service is ministered appropriately. The questionnaire should address this in detail and arrive at an accurate picture of the condition and its consequences for the client. This aspect can be uncomfortable for both parties, but nevertheless is an integral feature of communicating the appropriate information on a need-to-know basis.

The condition of the premises must also be assessed in order to establish any difficulties in moving around. Narrow passageways, steep stairs, lack of bannisters, bathrooms and toilets too small, and access to the premises are all contributory factors to the risks of the operation. Where the heating is inadequate, additional risks arise in cold weather.

Another factor to be taken into account is the presence of other family members. Although such home-care services are generally provided for clients living alone, this is not always the case. Where there are other family members inhabiting the same house, it is not uncommon that the health of such other members is also poor. Difficulties can arise in distinguishing who the client is, as the needs of other family members become apparent. Frequently, the health of one spouse has deteriorated to the point that the partner cannot be cared for as had previously been the case, and home care is being sought for this reason. Any potential care worker will have to keep in mind that the health of both spouses has a bearing on the outcome of the service. Giving relief to the resident carer is extremely important for the continued independence of the family unit.

Where the purchaser SSDs are undertaking the assessment, there is a programmed questionnaire for the assessment which, on completion, provides for a specific range of tasks that the service user and any family member can do, and so the services required of the agency care worker can be specified clearly. But not all SSDs are able to undertake such sophisticated assessments and they rapidly become out of date when the service user is very infirm. In such cases, the SSD requires the agency care worker to accept the assessment and perform the required tasks. This adherence to the contract specifications is considered as an absolute in the world of contracted services or goods, but may seem an inflexible attitude in the provision of the care, the purpose of which is to facilitate greater independence.

In block purchasing agreements, it is unlikely that the care agency will be formally introduced to each client, and the agency care workers are simply instructed to call at a number of addresses to undertake very specific tasks. This can lead to confusion in the mind of the service user, who will be forgiven for assuming that the agency care worker is a member of the SSD staff. This routine use of agency care workers, often undertaken when SSD staff are not available (for example, out of hours or during holidays), is not uncommon. Thus, any lack of familiarity with the service user and surroundings can lead to risks, especially where specialised equipment has been installed. If an agency care worker is not familiar with a service user's routine or their equipment, the time taken to complete the scheduled task may increase, possibly delaying the next assignment. In contracting with a private home-care organisation in these circumstances, the SSD staff must ensure that high-quality information is passed on.

Punctuality

Time and timing are central to the proper functioning of a care service, and this factor is the least controllable at the private agency. The concept of control is at the heart of most service-oriented organisations, and it would be stating the obvious to say that poor control is indicative of a poor service.

Generally, an employer can use an internal disciplinary procedure to reinforce his or her authority where an employee breaches work rules. Ultimately, there will be the threat of dismissal. But an agency generally cannot dismiss a person, even if a disciplinary procedure is available. Poor timekeeping need not always be the fault of the care worker, who may have been detained by an earlier client or simply have been caught up in traffic. Furthermore, the administration of most agencies will not take account of travelling time when scheduling timetables. However, this may change with new technology that tracks the movements of care workers, and the application of the Working Time Directive has obliged organisations who operate round the clock to review their working practices. The trend has been to overlook poor timekeeping, as most private clients and care workers develop good relationships.

Where SSDs purchase services, the issue of punctuality can be of greater significance and failings may be logged into a monitoring system, which will then be reviewed when the contract or accreditation period nears its end.

As the majority of agency care workers are female part-timers, who can easily get other work, removing unpunctual care workers from the register means that the agency will not be able to enlist that care worker for any future client. When new clients present themselves in the localities in which the care workers reside, the business principle to match the two is too great a temptation. Thus, removal of care workers from an agency's lists for reasons other than gross misconduct or criminal behaviour is unlikely.

Will the same care worker be attending all the time?

Private home-care providers will always try to keep a single care worker, or those already known, with a client or service user. SSD purchasers will often insist that the same person attends, and all home-care organisers know that clients feel deeply about a stranger visiting them.

It would be foolish for any business to offer a guarantee of the same person, and care agencies are only too familiar with the irritations and distress caused by the inability to provide a consistent service. Any client or service user should be informed that a new care worker is attending, out of courtesy, the need for safety and good business practice. Such communications build bridges between the client and the firm. This level of consistent service and effective communication are observable signs of quality.

Where a live-in service is provided, the identity of the care worker is fairly central to the contract, and the client and care worker should be allowed a face-to-face interview where possible, in order to determine compatibility. But this is not necessarily the rule. The Working Time Directive may affect the number of hours a live-in care worker will be available for work. Such workers may also be affected by the Minimum Wage legislation.

Is the care worker trained?

A good home-care provider will only use trained care workers and will display this information as a badge of quality. But the commercial pressure to use untrained care workers is very great indeed. The thoroughness and regular updating of care worker training are clear signs of quality in domiciliary care services and create a significant expense for any organisation.

There is a strict obligation to provide instruction in manual handling – sending a care worker on an assignment which could expose the care worker and/or client to risk of injury through manual handling could lead to a civil lawsuit and a criminal prosecution (Manual Handling Operations Regulations 1992) of the employer responsible for the care worker involved. Care workers are not only expected to undertake supposedly simple tasks, but should also be able to conduct themselves with composure and cheerfulness. Such a profile places certain demands on training, the following aspects of which rank as either essential or very important.

- **Transfers**: a large proportion of assistance provided by the home-care worker is to enable a client or service user to move from a sitting or lying position to some other position, often elsewhere in the house. There are specified ways of doing this, which may involve using a hoist when the movements of the client or services user are very limited. Hoists are now available in a variety of shapes and sizes, and can be controlled electrically. A new home carer should not attempt to use a different piece of equipment until he or she is completely confident with its operation. It is also important to be trained sufficiently to be able to judge whether or not the hoist is in good order.

- **Dealing with pain and discomfort**: as might be expected, clients with limited movement may be in pain all the time, or when being moved. A home-care worker should be in a position to deal with this prospectively, minimise discomfort and engage the client in some other way.

- **Cooking, hygiene and feeding**: limited mobility will mean that the client or service user cooks infrequently and is unable to do regular shopping. The home-care worker should anticipate the food stock and prepare food in an appropriate fashion, uncomplainingly. Feeding an adult requires as much skill and patience as feeding a child.

- **Skin care**: elderly or disabled people may have very delicate skin for many reasons, and the homecare worker must know exactly how to care for each type of skin.

- **Dressing, bathing and toiletting**: caring for another in such an intimate way requires enormous sensitivity and clear thinking, to maximise the comfort of the client or service user and to preserve his or her dignity.

- **Catheter care**: this should only be carried out by home-care workers with very specialised training, normally in a hospital or nursing home. Where this is required, a thorough risk assessment of the client's needs must be communicated to the home-care worker, who should be fully conversant with all aspects of client care.

- **Disposal of used incontinence aids and other equipment**: this aspect of care will provide positive clues to a visitor, as proper disposal leaves no traces.

- **Administration of medicines**: unqualified care staff are not usually required to minister medication, and where a client or service user takes medication in the presence of another, a home-care worker may record this, if necessary, in a record book kept for such purposes. Clients or service users who must take medication in order to remain at home – as opposed to being an in-patient – must not rely on a home-care worker to supervise this. It is unlikely that a home-care worker will have sufficient training to understand the consequences of side-effects or dosage variation, or be insured adequately to carry the liability.

- **First aid**: home-care workers should hold a current First Aid Certificate.

- **House cleaning**: this activity can be undertaken at varying degrees of intensity, and detailed instructions must be given.

- **Shopping and finance**: such work must only be given to those who are proven to be competent as well as trustworthy, and places clients or service users in a difficult situation if they have no relatives or close friends whom they can trust. Pension and benefits books should never be handed over to an assistant unless there has been prior agreement with the organisation and a protocol agreed (e.g. the book is only taken on a specific day to a specific post office, where hopefully the cashier will recognise the assistant). All transactions should be written down in the record book or receipts kept.

- **Bereavement counselling**: such special skills should not be rare, and the organisation's representative should be able to confirm the abilities of the home-care worker.

- **Liaison with visitors**: what communications are to be made to others should be clarified at the outset – during the assessment stage. If healthcare workers such as the district nurse attend, a certain exchange of information may be inevitable or essential. Any such communication should only relate to the care of the client/patient on a need-to-know basis. It may be important to communicate with other visitors, such as family members, and this must be discussed and clarified beforehand in order that a home-care worker confines herself or himself to appropriate communications.

The communication skills of the organisation's representative and the home-care workers will be critical in convincing a prospective client of the abilities of the home-care workers and the quality of the service. This list of training needs is not exhaustive and prospective purchasers of home care should make enquiries to ensure that claims made by organisations with respect to training are valid.

Is the care worker honest?

An agency offering a care service is exempt from the Rehabilitation of Offenders Act 1974 by the Rehabilitation of Offender (Exceptions) Order 1975, is free to request the prospective care worker to disclose all past criminal convictions and can ask the care worker to obtain a police check on her or his record. This will not inform the agency as to the honesty of a care worker, but will provide some clue and presumably deter convicted thieves. But most organisations cannot guarantee that a worker will never commit a criminal act, and obtaining care workers who are public spirited and caring is unusually difficult, for the reasons already mentioned. A home-care worker can also be in a vulnerable position with respect to a generous and forgetful client, and most care agencies insist that care workers must not accept gifts.

What checks are made on the care worker?

As well as police checks, good references are essential, and ideally the care worker will have held a position in the past so that a previous employer can speak for them. Reliable and dedicated workers are not commonplace and are often known in their localities. Such people often provide assistance to others on a voluntary basis and will have excellent references. The care agency will always make great efforts to check on the previous activities of care workers, and a considerable evaluation is made during the interview and induction of new staff.

Some firms insist on uniforms and badges, which provide a corporate image, and allow the care worker to be recognised. This is generally taken as a sign of quality and attention to detail.

Establishing reliability

A very difficult aspect of the job is the reliability of home-care workers in attending and working according to plan. The work is isolated, with little or no supervision, and conversation may be limited, depending on the client. The work may be repetitive or uninteresting, even boring. If the home-care worker is not entirely dedicated to the holistic care of the client, the various tasks that are required can seem like drudgery. This kind of care, when given by a family member, is generally regarded as sacrificial and heroic. It must be borne in mind that the majority of clients who require home care are not 'getting better'. Thus, the same home-care worker, calling regularly, week after week, is possibly witnessing a permanent decline of another person. In a hospital or nursing-home ward, comfort can be had from one's co-workers. It is indeed distressing to witness someone decline into severe helplessness.

Reliability is an uncommon attribute and is generally associated with stability and some kind of training. Such people often have strong beliefs in the desirability of the service user or client to remain within the home. This inner strength shows itself in their dedication to the work and their ability to strike up appropriate relationships, show respect and be respected. These 'marks' of reliability can usually only be evidenced by meeting such a home-care worker or through reports about them from other professionals and clients. It is remarkable that such people do consider that providing care is essential and part of their own vocation, as the pay rarely warrants this degree of dedication.

Improving quality

The problems attached to maintaining quality in delivering home care have been addressed by the recent Department of Health White Paper, *Modernising Social Services*,[2] in which the task of a regulatory system in social care is described in Chapter 4. There is an intention to create a General Social Care Council (GSCC), Commissions for Care Standards (CCS) and registration systems. Paragraph 4.22 provides that 'registration requirements will be uniform, regardless of whether the organisation is private, voluntary or statutory, and whether it is a "principal" organisation or an agency'.

Paragraph 4.23 refers to the registration of domiciliary care providers by their regional CCS if they meet the following criteria: fitness of owner or manager; personnel issues, including vetting and training; information provided to service users/clients; quality control systems; operational policies; and financial viability and insurance.

The issues of staffing and social services in general are addressed in Chapter 5 of the White Paper, recognising the huge increase in this employment sector – currently around 1 million people. 'People who work in social care are called on to respond to some of the most demanding, often distressing and intractable human problems'[2] (paragraph 5.2) and yet the vast majority of these workers have no recognised qualification or training. Additionally: 'the standards and suitability of some education and training in social care do not enjoy general confidence'[2] (paragraph 5.3).

In paragraph 5.5, the government proposes to 'develop a new training strategy centred around a new National Training Organisation for Social Care Staff'. This training organisation for personal social services will include in its functions, the identification of training needs and the ability to ensure that those needs are met.

References

1 Smith J (1998) Integrating the care of older people. *Croner's Health Service Manager Special Report* **18**.

2 Department of Health (1998) *Modernising Social Services*, Cmd. 4169. The Stationery Office, London.

6
Your rights if the standards are not met

All care agencies recognise that clients are put in a difficult position if they do not receive the service they were expecting and ought to expect. Where the organisation contracts with SSDs, a complaints procedure must be explained to the client and must also be available in writing so that it can be utilised at some point after the home-care worker has left. It should also be explained that the home-care worker is either self-employed or the employee of the client, depending on which of these relationships the agency has adopted. SSDs generally insist that the home-care worker is an employee of the agency, which must be fully insured, while undertaking work for SSD service users, in order that the SSD cannot be sued by the service user. Under the Trade Descriptions Act 1968, the agency is obliged to disclose these relationships.

The Department of Trade and Industry is informed of the abuse of the system by some organisations that fail to disclose their agency status to prospective clients, and is considering a root-and-branch reform of the law relating to agencies.

It is possible that the private organisation is offering a service, as opposed to staff for hire, which will be covered by the Supply of Goods and Services Act 1982, which provides in subsections 13–15, that the service must be provided with reasonable care and skill, within a reasonable time and that the charge that is levied must be a reasonable charge. It is important to recognise the implications of what has been said to the client – these are known as representations on which a person would rely. If a client has relied on a statement, either from the local authority or a care provider, about the nature of the service, and the statement turns out to be false, then a client may be able to take legal action against either or both if the outcome of that reliance caused a financial loss. In 1994, in a case concerning a childminder who had been recommended by a local authority officer, the court found the local authority and the officer in question liable for negligent mis-statement (*T* (*a minor*) v. *Surrey County Council and others* [1994] 4 All ER 577).

If a client is told that the same person will be calling at a specified time, and that turns out to be untrue, then the usual procedure is to complain. However, if the home-care worker is unavailable, then the only sensible thing would be to request another. The agency should inform the client of the problem and explain that another care worker will call. A good relationship will follow from good-quality communications and will prevent undue suffering. But if the home-care worker causes harm, either to the client or to the client's property, other remedies may be sought.

The agencies indemnify clients who might suffer harm through a home-care worker's acts while she or he is working. Thus, if the harm is caused at another time, then the indemnification may not be applicable.

Where an agency cannot meet its client commitments with its own care workers, it may wish to use the care workers from another agency. Most SSDs will not agree to this 'assignment' of the contract, and private clients should ensure that if such an assignment did take place, any insurance policy relating to the indemnification of the care agency was not invalidated.

A similar problem occurs when a care worker makes an unscheduled visit. If the client suffers harm on such an occasion, it is unlikely that any indemnity insurance will be valid. There are no cases reported, and it is difficult to speculate on the statistical incidence of such activities. Harm that is criminal in nature must be reported to the police and it should also be reported to the care organisation in question.

The standards relate to attendance, the unchanged identity of the care worker, their competence and their composure. The losses incurred by these failings will invariably amount to severe inconveniences rather than actual losses, but distress may be caused by unexpected new faces, and taking legal action might seem futile when the sums of money at stake are considered.

For the majority of service users, where the contract has been placed by SSDs with a private organisation, apart from following the complaints procedure there remains the option of taking legal action. But for the majority of such problems the financial losses flowing from a poor service would not warrant legal action, even if Legal Aid was available. For private clients who might suffer financially from, say, a failure to attend, then legal action in breach of contract or negligence may be considered. But the financial losses would need to be substantial, as mounting a case is not without its costs and stresses.

The greatest weapon in the hands of a dissatisfied client or service user is to refuse the service and, possibly, inform the press. Complaining to SSDs and the care agency may not yield significant improvements if there is an insufficiency of staff. But all organisations should at least have a monitoring system, of which complaints are only one component. There should be internal systems dedicated to collecting data on arrivals, departures and training levels, and this information can be used to substantiate claims of quality and complaints.

Creating charters is a common way for many public and private organisations to set a benchmark, giving the 'customers' a clear indication of what kind of service they can expect. Such charters may contain target numbers, such as the punctuality of the service. The passengers' charter for the train services is an example. Nevertheless, when failures occur, there are often insufficient remedies. A free ticket for a future trip may not actually resolve the problem of being late in the first place. Some care providers have produced charters for clients and care workers. Charters issued by care providers may contain statements such as '*Your dignity as a human being will be respected*' (UKHCA Code of Practice). Ideally, such charters should also contain a list of instructions on the steps to be taken if any of those statements are not fulfilled. It has been suggested that such statements can be construed as contractual terms, and that breach of the standards described therein is equivalent to a breach of contract. If the statements cannot be construed as conditions, as they do not go to the root of the contract, it is likely that they will be construed as a warranty. Breach of warranty has a lesser impact on the losses, and when proved, courts may award damages to the injured party. But bringing a case to court will need proof, and such statements, made with the best of intentions, will generally be difficult to substantiate.

Complaining to the Employment Agency Standards Inspectorate based in the DTI may bring about an improvement in the standards of conduct of a particular agency. The Inspectorate's Help Line is 0645 555105

Problems with services in general

Services provided by professionals such as solicitors, accountants, surveyors, banks, opticians and dentists tend to be easily accessible and the quality less uneven than in the past, although the final bill may be unexpected. There have been recent attempts to persuade such professionals of the need for transparent charging, clear statements about what the client can expect and full indemnification or professional liability insurance. The last of these is increasingly important, given the financial implications of the advice given and readiness to litigate when the advice fails. Most professions are regulated by statute or self-regulated in order to uphold standards. The fashion for charters is spreading, providing customers and clients with information about what they can expect, and what type of failure constitutes a failure that may be acted upon by making a formal complaint. Proving a breach of contract or making a claim in negligence are possible, as was demonstrated in *Midland Bank Trust Co Ltd* v. *Hett, Stubbs and Kemp* [1979] Ch 384, where a solicitor negligently failed to register an option for the purchase of land and the court held that the plaintiff could sue both in contract and in negligence. Such professions undoubtedly have assets and are heavily insured. The wronged client can effect redress without too much stress.

Services to the home

Most services to the home are bedevilled by the same problems of availability, quality and consistency. Obtaining a plumber, for example, can be a taxing if not vexing exercise. It is impossible to know if a plumber is free on the day you expect them, especially if he or she operates as a sole trader alone. Lack of secretarial staff means that booking can be difficult if a diary is not properly kept. The client is often on tenterhooks before and during the job of work. In spite of the efforts of self-regulation bodies, domestic services are not as easy to obtain as one might hope and are still prone to problems of quality.

Taking legal action in order to recover one's losses is not the easiest of undertakings. Tradespeople, and builders in particular, can adopt the 'escape hatch' of placing all physical assets in the name of a spouse or family member so that a successful litigant cannot denude them of assets. Obtaining redress through the courts will depend on the degree of loss incurred, but is not so readily obtainable.

> *Hoenig* v. *Isaacs* [1952] 2 All ER demonstrates the difficulties of paying for services which are not satisfactory. Mr H was taken on for redecoration and refurbishment of a flat, at the agreed price of £750.00. However, after he stopped work, Mr I only paid him £400.00, saying that as he had not finished the job, he should not have to pay the agreed amount. Mr H went to court, and Mr I was ordered to pay £350.00, less the cost of remedial work, estimated at £55.00.

In some services, typically package holidays, arbitration can be resorted to in the first instance to settle a dispute. This is commercial arbitration, governed by the Arbitration Acts 1950, 1979 and 1996. This must not be confused with the arbitration available in the small claims court of the county court, nor the procedures of industrial relations. It is a private, legally binding dispute resolution process, but is not necessarily a low-cost alternative to court. The arbitrator is someone who has some expertise in the relevant field of commerce and who has also trained as a commercial arbitrator, with organisations such as the Chartered Institute of Arbitrators in London.

Domiciliary care services

Such a range of difficulties applies equally to domiciliary care, in spite of the declarations of government spokesmen on availability of choice. In the free market that prevails in the availability of services, the levels of demand usually dictate the density of services likely to be found in a specific geographical area. For example, obtaining the installation of an intruder alarm system in a city will be easier than finding the service in a remote rural location. However, as the service includes the provision of goods of a reasonably high value, most suppliers will consider it to be worthwhile to travel to a remote location, and any extra costs will be included in the price.

Contractual relationship

There are a number of possible contractual arrangements in the domiciliary care sector.

Scenario 1

In a principal organisation (see p 19) the contract is between the care worker and agency. The client pays the agency the requisite fee for the service and the agency pays the care worker. Such a contract will be covered by the Supply of Goods and Services Act 1982, and the agency will be fully liable for the acts and omissions of the care worker while on duty. There is no contractual relationship between the client and the care worker.

Scenario 2

In the case where the agency acts for the care worker who is self-employed (*see* pp 19 and 20), there are two contracts, one between the client and the agency, and the contract between the care worker and agency. The client pays the agency the requisite fee and the agency pays the care worker. This fairly usual relationship may have some protection. The agency will be indemnified for claims against it through the acts and omissions of the care worker, but it is unlikely that the care worker will be indemnified in any way. Any financial losses incurred through injury at work may be uninsured. Although, technically, a client could sue the care worker for breach of contract, it may be more fruitful to sue the agency, which is indemnified and, also, may have some contributory liability in the breach.

Scenario 3

Where the agency acts for the care worker who is employed by the SSD or an individual (*see* pp 19 and 20), the contract between the care worker and agency relates to the commission charged for the introduction and placement. The employer pays the agency the requisite fee and employs the care worker. The agency drops out of the picture. The contractual rights will extend only to the task of introductions and placement. Thus, if, subsequent to a placement, the employer considered that the agency had failed in finding someone suitable or had transgressed in some other way, there may be a case for breach of contract or negligence.

Collateral contract with the agency

Thus, it is very important to know the actual status of the care worker. However, the vast majority of communications to arrange the service are between the client and the organisation, and in the event of a breach with serious consequences, it is unlikely that the agency will be able to hide behind the cloak of an introductory service. Under the Misrepresentation Act 1967, sellers are obliged to make accurate representations or statements about matters concerning the sale. Furthermore, anyone in the 'care' business would be expected to have wide knowledge of the significance of statements made with respect to providing care for a disabled person.

It is the central organisation, after all, that has made representations about the service and the quality of its care workers, and it would not be unusual for an agency to agree to provide a care worker for the client without actually knowing in advance who the care worker was going to be. In such cases, the courts can hold that a collateral contract exists, which is a contract running alongside the contract for services, and in which the agent incurs liability. Thus, if liability is incurred, the agency will bear the financial burden of the injured party's losses.

In order to make a claim for breach of contract, the client should have suffered some loss. Otherwise, without making a claim for damages – which is the quantification of the loss – the court is likely to award a nominal sum, which may not even pay for the expenses involved in litigation. Generally, damages are not awarded for emotional distress, anguish or vexation, but have been awarded when the object of the contract was to provide enjoyment or peace of mind.

> In *Jarvis* v. *Swan Tours* [1973] QB 233, [1973] 1 All ER 71 CA, the travel agent's brochure invitingly described a holiday 'as a houseparty in Switzerland' assuring that the customer would have a 'great time'. Mr Jarvis booked the holiday, paid the price and set off for the 'party'. To his astonishment, the hotel manager did not speak English and there were no other guests in the second week. Many of the descriptions in the brochure were simply not true. Mr Jarvis took the travel agents to court and won half of the amount that he claimed. Unhappy with this, he appealed for the full amount, and Lord Denning MR said that the loss of such an amenity could be recovered in damages, and that the statements in the brochure amounted to representations or warranties. 'If the contracting party breaks his contract, damages can be given for the disappointment, the distress, the upset and frustration caused by the breach'.

If, owing to the failure of the care worker, a client suffers a consequential loss, because an opportunity to do something has been lost, then this should be put to the care provider. An example might be that a home-care worker's visit enabled the client or another person in the household to visit a bank, or pay a bill or some other errand. When the visit from the home worker is crucial in this sense, it is essential to inform the office of the significance of the visit. It is likely that the terms and conditions of trading will include an exclusion clause for losses related to failure to attend. Some services are provided for a highly specific purpose, as shown in the following case.

> *Heywood* v. *Wellers* [1976] QB 446, [1976] 1 All ER 300 CA: Mrs H had

given instructions to Mr W, a solicitor, to obtain an injunction against a man who she feared. She wanted to prevent him harassing her. The solicitors neglected to obtain the enforcing injunction, Mrs H was molested as a result and suffered mental distress. She won damages in court for the molestation and the mental distress.

Lack of privity or contractual rights

When the SSD, or any other statutory organisation, purchases home care for the benefit of a service user, a triangular relationship arises. The contractual agreement is between the purchasing organisation and the home-care provider, and is validated by the consideration (a legal word for the money paid as the price) passing from the purchaser to the provider, who has been commissioned to provide care for a third party – the service user.

In this scenario, the service user or recipient of care has no contractual rights and is not privy to the contract even though they are a beneficiary of the contract, and if the contract is breached, the purchaser must sue the provider. This principle of English law is demonstrated below, and has been criticised frequently for its inflexibility.

> *Tweddle* v. *Atkinson* (1861) 1 B.& S. 393: In 1855, a father and father-in-law to be promised each other or contracted with each other to donate a sum to William Tweddle on the event of his marriage, as was the custom. They put this in writing, and included the right for the son to sue them. Before the gifts were made, the father-in-law had died. William sued the executor of the estate, but as he was only a beneficiary of the contract and not a party to it, he had no contractual rights.

The problem with this scenario, the SSD contracting for care for a service user, is that the purchaser would have difficulty in proving the losses suffered. The solution would be to take legal action on the basis of negligence. Negligence is a civil wrong and may or may not be related to a contract. It can be defined as the breach of a duty of care, and the person making the allegation of the breach, the injured party, would have to prove that a duty of care existed and that its breach caused the losses suffered. Contracts often provide for duties, as demonstrated below.

> *Donoghue* v. *Stevenson* [1932] AC 562: Mrs D and a friend visited Mr Minchella's cafe in Paisley. They ordered bottled ginger beer and ice cream. The friend paid. It was alleged that as the ginger beer was poured on the ice cream (a local delicacy), a decomposing snail

appeared, after which Mrs D suffered severe gastroenteritis. She had not bought the ginger beer, and so knew that she could not sue Mr M. She sued the bottler Mr Stevenson, on the basis that he had a duty of care to her. The case was a difficult one, covering a new legal principle, that of non-contractual negligence. It was held that such a duty of care did exist – that anyone contemplating an act had a duty to consider the risks involved to anyone who could be affected by that act, the so-called neighbour principle. This principle has been used repeatedly in the civil courts.

The plaintiff, i.e. the person who has suffered the wrong or loss, would need to establish that the care provider owed them a duty of care, and that the duty was breached and that the breach of the duty caused the loss. In order to establish whether or not a duty existed, and the nature of that duty, knowledge of what care providers usually did, and how they did it, would be necessary. In cases of professional negligence, the courts use a technique called the Bolam Test, to establish whether or not the standard of the duty of care was breached. The Bolam Test provides for a reasonably objective analysis of the kind of skill that a reasonable person could expect in those specific professional circumstances.

> The test is the standard of the ordinary skilled man exercising and professing to have that special skill. A man need not possess the highest expert skill; it is well established law that it is sufficient if he exercises the ordinary skill of an ordinary competent man exercising that particular art ... Negligence means failure to act in accordance with the standards of reasonably competent medical men at the time (*Bolam* v. *Friern Hospital Management Committee* [1957]).

Although there are very few cases of local authorities being held negligent in the discharge of their community-care duty, nurses who provide personal care to patients can be sued if their actions cause harm to the patient, e.g. scalding the patient in the bath. It is not a great leap in principle from being bathed by a nurse to being bathed by a care worker, who, one assumes, would be just as trained and conscious of the consequences of inattention to running a hot bath. The principle of *Donoghue* v. *Stevenson* is that of foreseeability.

Under the principle of vicarious liability, the plaintiff – the person who has suffered the loss and wishes to take legal action – would be able to sue the care provider, whether or not this is an agency or a direct provider. It is an established common law principle that one person or party may be held responsible for the negligent actions of another, usually through the relationship of employment. Although agencies may wish to disclaim the liability, it is unlikely that the legal representative and courts would limit themselves to suing an individual who is not likely to have any assets. Furthermore, the care-provider organisation, having been instrumental in providing the services of the individual in question, and having the responsibility of ensuring that care workers are adequately and suitably trained, would bear some if not all, the responsibility for the standard of their work.

Personal injury, which can include psychiatric injury, provides a strong ground for suing in negligence, and the courts will quantify the injury by awarding damages in a successful claim by an injured party. The damages are based on an assessment of the financial consequences of the injury, plus a component of the general damages which may be unquantifiable, such as pain and distress.

Intrusion of personal privacy

Engaging a person within one's home, on whatever legal basis, will mean an inevitable loss of privacy. Even if personal care is not required, activities such as shopping will necessitate the giving of information to someone else about one's personal habits. The home carer will undoubtedly be concerned about doing the best for the client, and will need to know about how to deal with emergencies. Giving consideration to these possible scenarios is not always welcomed, and providing names and addresses, details about medication, spare keys and any other personal details can bring about feelings of disempowerment. The more personal the care required, the more intimate details will be disclosed, generally unwillingly. The home care worker becomes less like a guest, entering at the client's behest, and more like the police. Furthermore, the more friendly a client or service user becomes with the care worker, the more information is divulged. Nevertheless, the care worker should be properly trained and will be alert to such feelings, and should be in a position to convey to the service user or client that all such information will be kept entirely confidential.

Equally, the care worker must not reveal intimate details about herself or himself, and must never chat about other clients, even if the other client is known to the present one. This is one of the more difficult aspects about providing training for care workers outside physical premises such as a hospital or nursing home.

Typical problems encountered

Punctuality and access to a client's house are the chief problems endured by service users and clients, but poor communication between the office and a care worker are the main cause of all the problems. The need for communication and travelling generally means that care workers must have a telephone and private transport. Such criteria are often obstacles to participation of some very well-intentioned people in a home-care service. People who may have spent years caring for a relative may find that that is their only occupational qualification and would be ideal as home-care workers. Lack of transport is frequently an impenetrable barrier to this kind of work if there are no clients nearby. Some organisations might provide either vehicles or transport for their care workers, and will consider this to be an efficient use of scarce resources.

One of the main problems encountered by agency personnel is the poor maintenance of confidentiality by the care workers. This is often attributed to the difficulties in training staff who have not had previous hospital or nursing/residential home experience.

When SSDs, or a private client, have purchased care for someone else, administration of medicines is often part of the daily routine. Unqualified staff are not usually permitted to administer drugs of any kind, and the purchasers and other residents within the house should bear this in mind.

Care workers taking a client out on a car journey should be insured, and most SSDs will include a term in the agreement that any such driver has business car insurance to include passengers. It is generally for the care provider to ensure that the care worker driver is fully competent and appropriately insured. It should be made clear from the outset that the client is capable of conducting him- or herself safely outside the home with the assistance of the care worker. Where a client or care worker uses a wheelchair, it must be established that the care worker is competent in dealing with any problems that might arise, and the trip will call for a high level of preparedness. Such assignments can be daunting for a care worker, and a well-trained person will demonstrate a mature attitude in preparing for such a trip.

When a client requires that the home-care worker drives the client's car, the provider should ensure that both driver and passenger are appropriately insured, and that the car is not of a type that the care worker is not qualified to drive. It will be the responsibility of the car owner to ensure the safety and roadworthiness of the vehicle.

How to complain

This can be an extremely difficult prospect for a client or service user. Those who have required care in the past may know only too well that getting a replacement might take some time, or that the complaint will inevitably affect the care worker, whom they have grown to like.

The relationship between a client or service user and the care worker can become close. In many circumstances, the care worker will be the person whom they see most often, or is the person who provides the most help in their lives. It is not uncommon for the client or service user to become friends with the care worker, and the sense of disappointment that can be experienced when the care worker moves on to another job can be deep.

Good care workers who are treated well by their 'employers', will tend to stay with the firm if they enjoy the job. But the work is poorly paid compared to some hospitals and nursing homes, and private well-heeled clients pay considerably more for the 'right' person. The alternative of working for one client alone, for several hours per week, may provide the right amount of security for many care workers, and even though they have proved excellent care workers to numerous clients in the past, the temptation to work in a more secure environment may well be too great.

Each care provider should include in their sales literature details of a reasonably simple complaint procedure. Where the organisation provides care for SSD service users, there are usually very straightforward procedures, which will be monitored by the quality control protocols of the SSD. If a SSD service user is in receipt of care from a private organisation, complaint should be made to both the care provider and the SSD. Making a complaint will not always rectify the situation, but should bring about improvement. When a care provider 'under contract' to a SSD has suffered many complaints, it may lose the SSD contract. But a private client need only terminate the contract with the organisation.

Generally, complaints can be made about specific failures in the delivery of service, such as poor timekeeping, rudeness, tasks left undone or unfinished, unsafe working practices, and so on. Where the care worker appears willing but incompetent, complaining can be more difficult.

Trained nurses or physiotherapists have recognised standards in their workmanship, and will belong to a professional association, whether they are working privately or in the NHS, which will keep them informed. Care workers will not always be in such a position, and the

lack of a recognised domiciliary care worker training standard and qualification means that the complaint of a client or service user may fall on
deaf ears.

The government has recognised this area of concern, and the independent Commission for Care Standards, proposed in the consultation
document *Modernising Social Services*,[1] will have responsibility for regu-
lating domiciliary social care providers, among other services. It is not
clear at the present time when such a regulatory system would be in
place.

The Department of Trade and Industry have also recognised this gap
in contractual liability relating to 'agency' staff, and have issued a
consultation on improving the regulation of employment agencies.[2]

Can you get your money back?

A private provider of care should specify in its literature how charges are
levied. This will normally be retrospectively for services rendered.
Generally, a timesheet is used, which is copied to care worker, client and
the office. This should provide an itemised statement of what services
were delivered, and the bill. Costs of these services are subject to VAT.
The client should keep his or her own copies of these documents, in case
of dispute. SSD service users, who are the recipient of services from a
private care organisation, paid for by the SSD, may not be provided with
such itemised statements, and each SSD will have its own procedure for
ensuring service delivery is logged and paid for in the manner prescribed.

Because SSDs are generally part of a larger organisation, the local
authority, the submission and payment of bills may proceed at a slower
pace, which can cause cash flow difficulties for the care provider.
However, where there has been a failure of service provision, the recti-
fication of contracts and billing can make a slow process even slower.

Cancellations: if the customer cancels

When a client cancels a visit, then the care provider may have to make a
charge, because the care worker concerned will not be able to get any
other paid work for that period. The client should note the necessary
amount of notice that should be given of a cancellation, as the care
worker may incur travelling expenses, which may not be recoverable.
SSD contracts may remain payable when the notice provided falls short
of the contract terms.

Cancellations: if the supplier cancels

With private clients, any cancellations should be agreed, and an aggreived client has the option of complaining or terminating the contract. No financial losses should be incurred. If a private client suffers repeat problems with different organisations, then he or she should seek advice from a neutral third party, such as a counsellor. When the new regulatory mechanisms have been implemented, more information on dealing with such problems will be available.

When a supplier cancels a visit requested by the SSD, then there could be a number of consequences, depending on the reason for the cancellation. The reason will often be staff shortages, but there may be mitigating circumstances, such as bad weather, sickness or, more foreseeably, Christmas holidays. Any combination of these could lead to a cancellation. As SSDs have contracted for these services in order to shift the risk and responsibility of providing their own staff to another organisation, such cancellations may be met with hostility. However, administrative staff who are inured to such problems will generally treat them phlegmatically. But private care providers will risk losing contracts they may value most dearly.

Where cancellations occur repeatedly for specific service users, both SSDs and the private providers should keep records and investigate any patterns that occur.

References

1 Department of Health (1998) *Modernising Social Services*, Cmd. 4169. The Stationery Office, London.
2 Department of Trade and Industry (1999) *Regulation of the Private Recruitment Industry: a consultation document*. The Stationery Office, London.

7
Health and safety

The objective of providing domiciliary care under the Community Care legislation is the maximisation of the independence of the individual as far as possible. This 'supported independence' at home inevitably requires a greater awareness of the risks to safety of people within the home environment. An accurate picture of the risks can only be obtained through an appropriate risk assessment, and the physical condition of the service user or client must be integral to this exercise, especially if any moving or handling is involved.

Recipients of funds under the Community Care (Direct Payments) Act 1996 and the Independent Living Fund are in a position to employ their own care staff, and so need to be especially aware of their general duty of care and their obligations under the Health and Safety legislation. An extension of the Direct Payments scheme has been proposed in the White Paper, *Modernising Social Services*, paragraphs 2.14–2.17. Section 2(b) of the 1997 Direct Payment Regulations (SI No 734) provides that any eligible person who appears to be capable of managing a direct payment by himself or with assistance can apply to be considered under the scheme. What is not clear is whether or not a care agency can be an instrument of 'assistance'.

The relevant local authority making the payments will be obliged to consider the capability of any qualifying individual and make a decision as to whether or not the applicant is capable, and if not, who may be in a better position to assist such a person. Certain categories of person, such as close relatives, are excluded by the Act from receiving payment for services. A care-providing organisation could be expected to have sufficient expertise in all the statutory obligations of a person employing a care worker and, if there is no conflict of interests, would be qualified to give such assistance. However, it is likely that it would not be considered as an impartial assistant, but rather, an organisation with a vested interest in selling its own services. Thus, recipients of grants and direct payments can find themselves in the position of being an employer. The

Health and Safety Commission (HSC) has undertaken a project to examine the position of care workers employed directly by a householder.

The requirement to be safe at work, and to keep one's employees safe, is governed by legislation, and the Health and Safety at Work etc. Act 1974 (HSWA) is the principal statute. However, section 51 provides that domestic employment is excluded, domestic premises being described as 'a private dwelling, including any yard, garden, garage or outhouse' as long as it is not shared by other non-occupants. There is no proposal to amend this exclusion of domestic servants, and it is important to note at this point that the majority of such employees will not be involved in personal care at all, but rather in general housekeeping and gardening duties. It is has been held that it would be too intrusive of personal privacy to impose legislation in such circumstances. Furthermore, drafting and enforcing such legislation would be exceedingly difficult.

In the face of creating an anomalous situation, it is more likely that a code of practice on good employment relations will be published – providing detailed guidance on all aspects of obtaining and keeping a care worker. The importance of the care assessment cannot be underestimated. Where SSD staff are involved in undertaking or commissioning care assessments, referral processes and monitoring, guidance provided by the Health and Safety Executive (HSE) should be adopted. In turn, the HSE should continue to contribute to the Department of Health's care management self-audit pack. This pack is for use by SSDs and health authorities (HAs) and provides information on health and safety.

The HSE will continue working on its health directorate project to produce guidance on practical solutions to manual handling problems in the community and, with the National Back Pain Association, to produce guidance on handling clients in the community.

Accidents and injuries

A considerable amount of home care is provided by organisations, and those who maintain an agency status will, irrespective of the claim that the care workers are self-employed, be responsible for ensuring that such workers are suitably trained. The same responsibility will lie with local authorities and healthcare providers. All community-care employers have a duty to their workers, whether or not the workers are on the employers' premises or those of the service user, patient or client.

The health and safety of both client or service user and care worker should be paramount, and the training provided should ensure that both are safe. The home of a client or service user is not controllable in the way that a workplace would normally be controlled by an employer. Visitors and other residents will have rights to enter and use the facilities. The knowledge of the home environment places a duty on any care agency to conduct their undertaking as carefully as possible.

Section 3(3) of the HSWA provides that employers and self-employed people have a general duty to give to persons who are not their employees, but who may be affected by the way the work is carried out, 'the prescribed information' about aspects of the work that might affect their health and safety. The Management of Health and Safety at Work Regulations also places on the agency a statutory duty to make a risk assessment before any undertaking, whether or not it is on the employer's premises. These statutory obligations are enforced through criminal sanctions.

The appropriate solution is for care providers to ensure, as far as possible, that all care workers sent to the homes of clients and service users are properly trained. Meaningful training represents a significant investment in each trainee, and the irregular nature of the work and the relatively low pay can act as disincentives to potential care workers. The problem areas are listed below.

Transferring a client

The vast majority of clients suffering from a moderate to severe disability will require assistance in transferring themselves from one static situation to another within the home, typically the armchair in the sitting room to the bed in the bedroom, or from a chair to the bathroom. If a wheelchair is used, invariably there are severe restrictions on space for turning the wheelchair and assisting the client at the point of transfer. These types of activities involve a degree of risk, which should be given consideration when the care plan is being drawn up.

The care worker should be fully trained in providing such assistance. Moving and handling injuries have formed a considerable proportion of work-related injuries in the past, and continue to do so. Regulations on moving and handling (Manual Handling Operation Regulations 1992 SI 1992 No 2793) provide limits on the weights that each individual should attempt to move and where two people or a mechanical hoist should be used. When a hoist is installed, its care and maintenance should be established, as it should for a wheelchair.

A related problem is the space required in a private home to install equipment such as lifts. The client may decide that a lift is required, but that no alterations – or no significant alterations – are made to the building. The consequences can be that at some later stage, when the client can no longer manage the transfer alone and assistance is required, there is inadequate space for the assistant.

Substances hazardous to health

When clients or service users have been running their own households, including gardens, for some considerable time before any assistance is required, it is not uncommon that chemicals, such as weedkiller or rat poison, have been stored in unmarked containers inside the house. This may have taken place some time in the past, when the client or service user was more active. Any hazardous substances must be treated with great care, and a new care worker will not make use of such containers, even if the client requests it.

More common substances include bleach, caustic soda, the various modern cleaning agents on the market and numerous solvents. Some suppliers provide information or data sheets on their chemical solutions. Care workers should be trained to recognise types of domestic cleaning substances and take the appropriate precautions.

Where incontinence care is integral to the care plan, disposal of biological waste must also be attended to in the proper manner. This may require a dedicated disposal system, which has to be collected on particular days.

The care agency may provide protective gloves and other clothing. A point of note is that a uniform, worn as part of the corporate image, does not constitute protective clothing.

Infections

It is usual for care workers to be immunised against hepatitis B, as it is the most easily transmitted of infectious diseases, although not especially common in the community. However, methicillin-resistant *staphylococcus aureus* (MRSA), a micro-organism that lurks in hospital wards, on the skin of certain individuals and inside some surgical wounds, cannot be immunised against. Any care workers attending clients or service users who are known to be infected by this organism must employ good barrier-nursing techniques. It is not unknown for a patient to be discharged from hospital suffering from an MRSA infection, usually in a wound. But, more likely, a patient will be discharged and remain a carrier. Only nursing staff should deal with such a wound, as MRSA is a communicable disease, but care workers should know about the care for such a client or service user.

A modern ethical dilemma is whether or not care workers should be informed of a client's or service user's condition, such as HIV status, AIDS or other sexually transmitted disease. However, it has been suggested that if proper infection-control techniques are learned and practised, then all risks are being attended to in the most appropriate fashion.

Electrical safety

The care workers are guests in the home of the client or service user, but nevertheless are entitled to be safe when using appliances, and will have a duty to act safely when caring for the client or service user. Where wiring is frayed, or where plugs and sockets are damaged, the care plan should include notice of such hazards and the care workers will not make use of them. Safety product suppliers should be contacted for lists of detector and protector appliances, which can be used to keep the operator safe.

Fire safety

Even in the late 1990s, it is possible for clients or service users to have open coal fires and no central heating. Fire precautions are difficult for a non-householder to manage, as they are intimately bound up with the premises and way of life of the client or service user. Smoking in an armchair or bed is not unusual, and a care worker is not in a position to frown upon it. Great difficulties arise when the smoking client or service user has a mental disability, and the care manager must give this special consideration. The care plan should include the observation of smoke detectors and alarms, and any special factors related to maintaining fire safety.

Physical environment

Care workers may dislike the fact that they must endure a smoking environment, but they are guests of the client or service user and must decline the assignment if they have strong feelings about smoking.

The condition of the premises is of concern to any domiciliary care provider. Not infrequently, a client or service user will have recourse to social services because of neglect of their personal selves as well as their property. Repairs may take some time, but vital personal care may be required immediately and, on occasion, this may need to be provided on the premises if a respite place in a nursing home cannot be found. It is for the care manager to assess the risks involved, but the care worker's safety must not be jeopardised.

A duty under section 4 of the HSWA may also apply to any common parts of a building, such as stairs and lifts, even though they are not used exclusively for occupation (*Westminster City Council* v. *Select Managements Ltd* [1985] 1AER 897).

Food hygiene

Care workers can be placed in delicate situations if required to prepare a meal for a client or service user when there is no food in the house. They should be trained in the hygienic preparation of food, and in using aids when necessary to assist in feeding. The shelf-life of the food in the house may be a matter of note, and it is therefore in the interests of all concerned that the same care worker attends the client or service user as far as possible.

Sharps

Any needles or blades must be disposed of appropriately in a hard container. They are a common cause of injury.

Assaults and challenging behaviour

The safety of both client or service user and care workers must be ensured. Care workers travelling alone at night in 'rough' districts can become a target and must take suitable precautions, such as travelling in pairs, using mobile phones, pagers or personal alarms. Violence in the workplace is not an uncommon occurrence within hospitals, and considerable research efforts are being made on the optimum ways of reducing violent incidents. Thus, an employer in the care business will be alert to risks of physical abuse faced by workers, whether or not they are on the employer's premises.

Where the client or service user exhibits challenging behaviour, the care agency must ensure that only care workers with appropriate mental health training are sent and that sound strategies are followed. Such care workers should always be able to maintain contact with the office.

Working Time Directive (WTD)

The new regulations, in force from 1 October 1998, provide for limits on hours per week, special health assessments for night workers and a minimum of 3 weeks paid holiday per year, rising to 4 weeks in 1999. For some care agencies, this will substantially increase the costs of providing a home-care service, and where a care worker works for more than one agency, it will be difficult to establish their total eligibility for leave, as a 'week' will depend on their average number of hours worked in a single agency.

Chapter 1 of the Regulatory Guidance from the Department of Trade and Industry (DTI) defines a worker; the majority of agency workers will be 'workers' for the purposes of the WTD and, in general, the employer of a worker will be obvious. For agency workers, the employer will be determined by the contractual arrangements, and where this is not possible, it will be whoever pays the worker.

The hours limit is 48 hours per week, averaged over 17 weeks, which may be extended in certain circumstances. Where a worker has more than one job, employers are required to take all reasonable steps to ensure that workers do not exceed an average of 48 hours per week. Thus, employers in care agencies would need to enquire whether the care worker was working elsewhere. There will be a need for accurate record keeping.

With respect to travelling, 'Time spent travelling to and from a place of work is unlikely to be working time as a worker would probably neither be working nor carrying out their duties. A worker may well be doing both if they are engaged in travel that is required by the job.' Generally, a guide would be that where the employer pays travelling expenses, the travelling time could count as working time.

Where the care worker is technically a domestic servant under section 51 of the HSWA, special considerations will apply. Generally, the hours limits will not apply, but entitlement to rest breaks, rest periods and annual leave will apply. The rest breaks are:

- 20 minutes between 6-hour periods of work

- 11 consecutive hours between each working day

- 24 uninterrupted hours in each 7-day period – which can be averaged over a 2-week period.

Daily and weekly rest are separate entitlements and in addition to annual leave.

This places live-in care workers in a difficult position, as they may not be able to incorporate breaks in a working day and may not be able to have a period of rest after a 48-hour working week. An assessment for each assignment would need to be undertaken with respect to night-work, which would entitle them to their own health assessments. Night-time is defined as a period of at least 7 hours including the period of midnight to 5 a.m. Unless there is a contractual term which specifies otherwise, it will 11.00 p.m. until 6.00 a.m. A night worker is defined as any worker whose daily working time includes at least 3 hours of night-time, on the majority of their working days, or on such a proportion of the days they work as is agreed between them and the employer, or sufficiently often for them to be described as night workers.

Chapter 3.1.4 of the Regulatory Guidance from the DTI provides for measures to be taken with respect to special hazards, or heavy physical or mental strain, the periods for which should not exceed 8 hours per working day. The length of the working week is the night worker's normal hours, and if the worker contracts to work overtime, then this is not normal working time. The calculations of night work are to be found in Chapter 3.1.7. Night workers are entitled to a free health assessment, with opportunities for further assessments at regular intervals. It is for the employer to devise a suitable health assessment. A screening questionnaire, compiled by a suitably qualified person who knows about the nature of the work, could be used, and should be updated regularly.

It is possible for a worker and employer to agree to contract out of these provisions. This should be in writing, and the worker must be allowed to bring the agreement to an end. The period of notice for terminating the agreement is 3 months (Chapter 2.2.1).

Reporting of accidents and injuries

A well-run care provider will have instituted a proper system of reporting accidents that concern staff, including care workers, and clients. Where contracts with SSDs are in place, the SSD may dictate the accident-reporting system. Submission of accident and incident data may form part of the accreditation procedures. Very few data are published on this aspect of home-care provision, and questioning staff at the care agency may not yield much information if they have only worked there a short time. Nevertheless, any care provider should be able to indicate their own statistics when required to do so.

Under the Reporting of Injuries, Diseases and Dangerous Occurrences Regulations 1995, if a self-employed worker is injured and cannot work for more than 3 days, then the controller of premises/employer is responsible. The HSE provides a useful guide, which includes reporting forms.

Duty of care on customer as householder

An occupier or controller of domestic premises has a statutory duty under the Occupier's Liability Acts 1957 and 1984 to ensure that invited visitors are safe, and that trespassers or unlawful visitors are also unharmed.

Section 2(1) provides that the duty is to take such care as is reasonable to see that the visitor will be reasonably safe. Thus all clients or service users will owe a duty of care – identical to the duty owed in common law negligence – for the safety of their care workers. The liability might be joint with another owner, such as a landlord. The duty extends to the safety of the care workers while they are doing what they are contracted to do.

Section 2(3)(b) of the 1957 Act provides that 'An occupier may expect that a person, in the exercise of his calling, will appreciate and guard against any special risks ordinarily incident to it, so far as the occupier leaves him free to do so'. Thus, if they are injured while in a part of the premises that they have no permission to enter, then the duty may not apply.

The reported cases include window cleaning, and liability has been shared between the occupier and the employer (*King* v. *Smith* [1995] ICR 339) where the window cleaner fell from a sill and was injured, and the employer only (*General Cleaning Contractors Ltd* v. *Christmas* [1952] 2 AER 1110) where the window cleaner was injured after a rotting sash fell on his hand causing him to lose his grip. He attempted to sue the occupier as well, but failed. Insurance against this type of legal action is readily available, often sold with house buildings insurance.

In the process of delivering care, the people attending may have to undertake risky manoeuvres, and if injury occurs and the injured party takes legal action, a good deal will depend on the foreseeability of the risk and attributable skill of the 'visiting worker'. In the case of *Neame* v. *Johnson* [1993] PIQR 100, an ambulanceman was injured while attempting to carry the unconscious occupier in a chair. The stairs were said to be poorly lit, and the ambulanceman knocked over a pile of books stacked by a wall on a landing, slipped and injured himself. The court held that the pile of books did not constitute a 'reasonably foreseeable risk of injury', and so the occupiers were not held liable for the ambulanceman's injuries.

Cases such as this place greater emphasis on the need for such self-employed workers to have personal accident insurance.

Duty of care on supplier

Under the Employment Agencies Act 1973, a care agency has a statutory duty to ensure that any staff being placed with a client are suitably trained. The agency will also have a duty of care when taking on a client and matching them with a care worker to ensure that any work being undertaken is safe for all concerned.

A client's home is not a workplace in the technical sense. It cannot be controlled by an employer, and the HSWA does not apply to a category of worker – section 51 provides that the Act will not apply to an employer of a domestic servant, nor to the servant in a private household.

But self-employed people have a statutory duty under section 3(2) of the 1974 Act to take care of their own health and safety, and employers (this will include organisations who subcontract work to self-employed people) have a statutory duty under section 3(2) to conduct their undertaking in such a way as to ensure, so far as is reasonably practicable, 'that persons not in their employment but who may be affected are not exposed to risks to their own health or safety'.

When constructing a care plan, all factors affecting the delivery of care should be taken into account. Care providers will generally use a checklist, and the representative – perhaps a care manager – will tour the premises and establish that the flooring, handrails, appliances, etc. are safe. This can be disconcerting for the occupier, but, nevertheless, the agency is under an obligation to know of any risks to the care worker. Ultimately, if the safety of the care worker is at risk, so also will the safety of the client or service user be put at risk. The physical premises, fixtures, fittings and appliances must be sound, and supplies of gas and electricity must also be in a good state of repair. The external premises, which are often in the domain of a landlord, commonly give cause for concern and so access and egress may need special attention. Where a care worker is required to accompany a client or service user on a journey, wheelchair or pedestrian safety requires special attention.

Many clients and service users do not live entirely alone – there may be other residents in the household or occasional visitors. A care agency is unlikely to obtain any undertakings from such people if they are not already involved in caring for the client. The generality is that the other residents will all be caring for the client at some point during the day – the care worker may be engaged in order that such carers have some respite. Where other residents are unresponsive, the agency and the care worker must assess whether or not the presence of such a person poses a risk.

Some care agencies will supply their care workers with personal safety alarms or pagers in order that their movements can be logged periodically. Good safety training is essential, and many lone workers are unaware of the risks.

Insurance

A care agency will have public liability insurance, third party liability insurance and employer's liability insurance to indemnify the organisation against claims from clients, members of the public and the employees. This last category will also include self-employed care workers. Some organisations offer accident and loss of earnings insurance to the care workers, as part of their remuneration, but it is more common for care workers to have to insure themselves.

If agency care workers are injured through work, they may not always be fully compensated for loss of earnings if they have not taken out adequate insurance, which is relatively costly. Statutory sick pay is a benefit payable depending on one's National Insurance history. In the light of the fact that many women take up part-time work as intermittent care workers, few will have recourse to any income if they cannot work.

Meaning of agency status

This is a curious grey area with respect to employment status. It offers embryonic enterprises the opportunity to increase or decrease their staffing levels without infringing employment statutes, and also the opportunity for new workers to get a feel for the type of work that may be of interest to them.

Agencies supplying secretarial, industrial and catering staff are well known, and can offer the services of secretaries and other staff who may be between permanent jobs, may prefer occasional work, may be in the country temporarily, or students during the holidays, and so forth. Agencies fill a gap in the market of supply and demand and so are able to sustain this no man's land status, governed by the Employment Agencies Act 1973.

But with respect to health and safety, the courts have judged the 'employer' to be liable for injuries sustained by 'self-employed' workers, undertaking projects for the contractor employer.[a] The DTI, in recognition of the fact that the Employment Agencies Act 1973 may need updating, has produced a consultation document, the aims of which are to bring about clarity on all sides of the role of the 'agent'. A significant aspect is the contractual relationships which are currently purported to be in force, but are not always explicit to the client. It is likely that any worker who cannot be described as truly independent will be deemed to be in contract with the bureau that arranged the work.

Responsibility for training

Any organisation purporting to offer care services must ensure that the care workers provided are properly trained. This can be done either through providing the training themselves, or by only taking on care workers who are already trained.

Some agencies will only take on care workers who have worked within an NHS hospital or a nursing home in the recent past. Such experience can mean that the care workers have worked with other professionally qualified staff and will have sound knowledge, not only of care techniques, but will also have communication skills and an understanding of an ethical framework. These last two areas of training are difficult to transmit in the short period given up for training agency care workers.

On first joining a care agency, a thorough induction should be carried out, and this will assist the office staff and management to evaluate the new care worker. References must be checked, but if the care worker has not worked recently, then a skill refresher course might be necessary. Providing the initial and ongoing training for the care workers allows

[a]*Lane* v. *Shire Roofing Co (Oxford) Ltd*, (*The Times* 22 Feb 1995), where a contractor asked a self-employed roofer to finish a specific job, and who was injured; *McMeechan* v. *Secretary of State for Employment*, where the court held that an agency worker might be an employee of the agency.

social interchange and gives the trainers a chance to see for themselves the skills of the 'operatives', who work largely unsupervised. The isolated and fragmentary nature of the work means that care workers rarely have opportunities to discuss training issues with qualified trainers.

The majority of training available is to improve moving and handling techniques. Assisting people with poor mobility within the confines of their own home can be fraught because of the restrictions of space. Furthermore, the regulations on moving and handling have been amended, and the 'employer' has a statutory duty to update the training and skills. The general purpose National Vocational Qualification Level 2 course in social care is a useful standard if an organisation does not have its own training and assessment programme. The NVQ route means that all and any relevant training is taken into account when awarding the certificate. However, it is important to validate that the training has taken place, and this should normally be done during paid time and at a time convenient for the care workers. An informal gathering of a trainer and a few care workers is an excellent opportunity to impress the care workers with the importance of an ethical framework, as well as providing 'core' information and discussing issues of importance to the care workers and the firm.

Assessment of the skills of the care workers should be conducted 'in the field'. An assessor may accompany a care worker on her or his assignment and record that specific tasks are done in accordance with the training protocols. This practical type of assessment is generally held to be much more appropriate than providing written scripts during an examination, and the NVQ system is designed to minimise the amount of writing that a candidate has to do.

8
Buying care for someone else

It is not uncommon for a family member to want to buy home care for another member of the family who is disabled or frail. This is most commonly an offspring for an ageing parent or, sadly, a spouse for the partner. Where this is being contemplated, it is vitally important to consult with the disabled member that the service is required. A carer, that is a person who normally cares for the disabled member, can become exhausted or poorly when looking after the disabled member, and this situation can become so serious that either or both are admitted to hospital, one for respite care and the other to recover their health.

For the avoidance of confusion, in this chapter, the person who is looking after or caring for someone will be described as the carer and the person who is being cared for will be described as the subject.

In circumstances where a family member is a carer, the SSD and the GP should be informed. Such carers now have a statutory right to be considered under the The Carers (Recognition and Services) Act 1995, but this has been implemented in a piecemeal fashion. The kind of exigencies endured by this group of approximately 6 million people are known to the Carers' National Association, who have produced a booklet in conjunction with the British Medical Association, *Understanding Caring*, in the Family Doctor series (obtainable from Family Doctor Publications, 10 Butcher's Row, Banbury, Oxon OX16 8JH). Such a publication is extremely useful for any individual or health professional who wishes to obtain home care for another person.

The type of relationship between the subject and the care worker is not one that fits easily into the present ethical framework. Although it is intended to serve a therapeutic purpose, it is not a therapeutic relationship, as the care worker is not in a position to offer advice. Neither is the care worker trained to perform any invasive techniques. Rather, the relationship is task based, and more closely resembles that between a 'master and servant', the manner in which employment relationships were described in the nineteenth century. This contractual relationship is, nevertheless, subject to overriding ethical principles related to the exercise of the subject's free will.

The individual who requested the care service, and who may be paying the bill, is the person in a contractual relationship with the care provider. The subject will be the beneficiary of the contract, as well as the individual who is paying, if the presence of the care worker offers some relief from the daily routines of caring tasks. However, where disputes have occurred, the courts have been ambivalent about such beneficiaries accruing legal rights of their own, as demonstrated below.

> *Jackson* v. *Horizon Holidays Ltd* [1975] 1WLR 1468: this case is similar to that of Mr Jarvis in Chapter 6, except that here, Mr Jackson bought a package holiday for himself and his family. The holiday did not turn out as described in the brochure and he won damages for himself only. He appealed to the Court of Appeal and Lord Denning MR stated that Mr Jackson 'should be able recover the expense to which they have been put ... he should also be able to recover for his discomfort, vexation and upset which the whole party have suffered by reason of the breach of contract ...'. However, the original damages were not increased.

The subject of the contract may have no contractual rights, but the care worker has a legal duty of care to act in such a way as to cause no harm, whether it is physical, psychological or emotional.

There are good reasons to adopt the principle that the care worker is assisting the carer, and that it is the carer who is the client. The tasks may involve the subject, but the objective of the care worker is to assist the client as far as possible, which may include sitting with the subject in a 'guardian' capacity, to enable the carer to leave the premises. This relationship may give rise to the least objection and leaves the carer in 'full charge' with respect to communicating with the subject. The care worker will also have no doubts as to her or his role, as long as the subject does not raise any objections to her or his assistance.

Consent

Whether or not home care is appropriate is a matter that can only be addressed by the recipient of the care. In a shared household, it may well be that the carer feels that some home help is essential in order that she or he has fewer tasks to do. Such extra help may provide opportunities for rest, going out, spending more time communicating with the disabled member of the family and so on. It is likely that most disabled individuals will welcome or accept the need for help, and acquiesce to any requests, in order to accommodate the carer. Where the disability is serious, there is some likelihood that the subject may be less likely to understand this need and possibly less likely to acquiesce to any requests.

In this context, the carer is often exhausted and the help required is for personal care of the subject. It is useful for the carer to obtain expert help, such as the district nurse or GP, in order to communicate fully the need for this home care to the subject. No one likes the thought of strangers in their home, and the more disabled a person is, the less wholesome is the thought of such a person entering their home and private personal space. The intimate nature of such help, and the help-lessness of a person suffering, for example, a stroke or terminal condition such as multiple sclerosis, renders the situation extremely sensitive.

In such situations, before contacting a care provider, it is useful to discuss the matter with the primary healthcare team members, such as the nurse or doctor most familiar with the subject, or any other person connected with the subject's well being, such as the local parish priest. The BMA and RCN have produced a useful booklet on this difficult topic, *The Older Person: Consent and Care* (1995).

If the plan to obtain care goes ahead, it is essential that the care worker enters the house as a welcome guest and the subject does not offer any objection to her or his presence. Such an objection is awkward for care workers to deal with. They are not trained nurses and have no profes-sional 'power and influence' such as that wielded by a nurse or physiotherapist.

Where personal care is being delivered, then the carer should not leave the care worker and subject alone together until the carer is satis-fied that the subject is consenting and co-operating where possible. This scenario indicates the importance of a regular and reliable care worker. There are legal outcomes if the subject is compelled to be 'handled' against their will: 'Every mentally competent adult has an inviolable right to determine what is done to his or her own body'.[1]

Putting an individual in fear of their safety or exerting any force on them constitutes assault and battery, and provides the subject with grounds for an action in trespass against the person. It is the same prin-ciple as trespassing on someone else's land. However, if the circle of people familiar to the subject have known about and understood the need for the care service, then such claims may be mitigated. The current law does not provide for an acceptable method of delegating powers and responsibilities for an adult to another adult.

Where the subject has a mental disability, the diagnosis of the mental condition does not necessarily mean that their powers of consent can be overridden. This is an ongoing ethical dilemma, exacerbated by the fact that many people suffering from a mental disability live in the community. However, the mental health teams will be fully aware of all the attendant problems and will decide on the delivery of personal care.

But the power of consent need not be overriding or total. That is to say, the law only requires the capacity to consent for the particular act in question. So, for example, when a very elderly man, having suffered a stroke, remarries and then executes a new will on the same day, he can be held mentally competent to marry, but not to make the will (in the Estate of Park [1954] P. 112).

Where the subject is elderly and mentally infirm, then the care manager must be fully aware of the subject's general feeling towards the prospect of a home-care service, and such services should be under supervision as they are likely to present with greater risks than clients or service users who are less disabled. It is common for a family member to take charge of such a subject's finances under an Enduring Power of Attorney (EPA), but as yet there are no such powers for taking charge of their personal welfare.

The Court of Protection is designed to protect the interests of patients who have become 'incapable by reason of mental disorder of managing and administering his property and affairs', by appointing a receiver for a patient. This person becomes, in effect, a statutory agent with the necessary powers written in the order of appointment issued by the Court or the Public Trust Office. By virtue of the Mental Health Act 1983, the Court can authorise any transactions necessary to maintain the patient, his family and dependants, and the Official Solicitor is a government-appointed watchdog over these affairs. The types of cases dealt with at his office cover many categories of litigation, affecting financial rights and personal injuries, as well as 'declaratory proceedings in the High Court and medical treatment decisions'. The Secretary of State for Social Security also has powers to appoint adults – individuals or organisations such as local authorities – to act on behalf of a claimant who, through mental incapacity, is unable to manage his or her own affairs.

However, there remain problems of incapacity to consent over one's personal physical care. The background is the demographic change in age structure and the fact that dementia will affect 5% of the population over the age of 65, rising to 20% in those over 80 years old. This aspect of decision making in adults was examined by the Law Commission during 1991–93. The present government, recognising a clear need for reform, has now issued a Consultation Paper, *Who Decides? Making*

Decisions on Behalf of Mentally Incapacitated Adults.[2] The deadline for responses was March 1998. A few salient points are referred to here.

The starting point proposed is that all adults are presumed capable of consenting unless proof to the contrary is offered, and this capacity is to be defined through a 'functional approach' (para. 3.6). It mirrors the case described above, which provides that a person may have capacity to determine some things but not others. Thus, an observed incapacity over a single matter will not necessarily mean that the subject has no capacity at all. The Law Commission, supported by the government, rejected the linking of the test of capacity with the concept of 'mental disorder'. But as to the question of communicating a decision, as well as the capability to make the decision itself, the Law Commission recommended a similar approach. If a person, whether capable of making a decision or not, could not communicate that decision because of unconsciousness or any other reason, then they could be held as not having capacity. The capacity to make a decision can be further defined as the inability to understand or retain the information relevant to the decision, or the inability to make a decision based on that information.

'The Law Commission has suggested a Code of Practice for the guidance of those assessing whether a person is or is without capacity to make decisions' (para. 3.16). In order to assess a person's decision-making capacity, the Law Commission proposed that all practicable steps, including explanation using other methods, should be taken to establish capacity first, and only when there is a failure can a person be deemed not to have capacity for that particular matter. A person should not be deemed as having no capacity just because the decision they made was not one that a prudent person might make. This approach could lead to inconsistency of application without further guidelines.

It goes without saying that when it is established that a person lacks capacity, those who do decide must act in the best interests of the mentally incapacitated adult. This could be measured by :

- establishing the past and present wishes of the person, including the factors that they may take into account

- encouraging the person to participate as much as possible, or improving their ability to participate in any decision

- consulting with other relevant people who would know the person's feelings on the matter in hand

- attempting to make the decision in question in another way – causing fewer restrictions on the person's freedom.

There is recognition that many informal decisions are already being made for those with limited or diminishing capacity, and that many carers, with possibly the best of intentions, are using an authority that may be 'unregulated in terms of protecting the person without capacity and poses a certain amount of risk for the carer in that they may have little or no legal basis for their action' (para. 3.26).

The Law Commission wished to uphold this informality of decision making, and wished to provide adequate legal protection for carers caring for those without capacity. It proposed that it should be lawful 'to do anything for the personal welfare or health care of a person who is, or is reasonably believed to be, without capacity in relation to the matter in question if it is in all the circumstances reasonable for it to be done by the person who does it' (para. 3.28).

The Law Commission also proposed that existing rules on contracting with people who lacked capacity should remain, which means that purchases for 'necessaries' should be charged at a reasonable price. Thus, persons without capacity can be provided with the basic goods and services. Further proposals were that a carer might pay using the money of the person without capacity; or pay first and claim the money back; or promise on their behalf to pay later. The government accepts these in principle – but is concerned about abuse.

On the basis of an EPA, empowering another named adult to exercise control of the subject's finances, the Law Commission has considered a Continuing Power of Attorney (CPA), which empowers another named adult to exercise control over personal and healthcare matters, property and affairs, including the conduct of legal proceedings. Just as with an EPA, the subject will empower another person at a point when they have capacity to do so. But concern has been expressed about the legitimacy of the 'proxy' in healthcare matters, which is not different to the problems associated with the implementation of an advance statement. The power must be transferred to another, at some point in time, in anticipation of diminished capacity. At what point in time is a decision about the future – usually unforeseeable – the current will of the subject?

The proposed legislation on these immensely significant topics will inevitably generate an intense philosophical, ethical and political debate.

Occasionally, a client or service user will have discharged themselves from an institution prematurely and may either buy the care service for themselves or it is requested by a family member. When erratic behaviour is displayed and the services of the care worker are refused after the care worker has arrived, then, unfortunate as it may be, the care worker cannot override the client or service user's decision. Whether or not that service remains unpaid will be a local matter.

There are powers under section 47 of the National Assistance Act 1948 for SSDs to compulsorily remove people from their homes, to a place of safety, because they are suffering from grave chronic disease or are physically incapacitated and living in insanitary conditions.

Advance statements

Making a decision about future treatment in advance is becoming more fashionable, and the government fully supports the rights of a patient to receive information about a proposed course of treatment, which the patient is entitled to refuse.

Consider the following scenario: a client or service user has been diagnosed with a terminal condition and is already disabled and poorly. A decision is taken to remain at home among familiar people and objects and let nature take its course. No intervention of any kind is to be made, especially the emergency services. Care workers attend for a few hours a day. Typically the care plan will require some food to be prepared, or to assist the client or service user in rising from or going to bed.

The care-providing organisation will have spent a considerable time in constructing its policies and rules about how the care workers conduct themselves, and what to do in the course of an emergency. Allowing a client or service user to remain unconscious will not be consistent with the policies of the care agency. When a care worker perceives an emergency, the training will dictate that the emergency services are called. Resuscitation is not usually part of the care workers' training.

Generally, resuscitation is regarded as an intervention, and may be proscribed by the individual. Where clients or service users do have such views about their own treatment, then it is useful to bear in mind that many volunteer helpers, health professionals and agency care workers will have difficulty in coping with such a plan if there is one. Obtaining advice from a hospice may be a solution. The British Medical Association has produced a *Code of Practice on Advance Statements* for health professionals and, in collaboration with the Patients' Association, has also produced a guide for patients about advance statements.

The need for terminal care is increasing, and it is likely that there are care providers who will specialise in this sort of case. Certainly, the legal position is that advance statements are currently binding at common law. The consequence of this is that an individual or company who infringes this wish could face legal action.

Importance of communication

The present government has agreed that the present situation with respect to the care of vulnerable people is unsatisfactory, as described above. The proposal to introduce regulatory mechanisms into social services, which can provide national guidance and codes of practice, will be welcomed by practitioners in the field. The discussion in this chapter will reinforce the need for wide consultation when there is universal acknowledgement of the need for another adult to have the benefit of social care services. Care managers, social workers and care workers may not assume that a subject who is not demonstrative is consenting. Nevertheless, there will exist a professional duty to act in the interests of the client or service user, and this must be done with great sensitivity and care. The need for well-qualified staff in mental health care is paramount.

References

1 Brazier M (1992) *Medicine, Patients and the Law*. Penguin, London.

2 Lord Chancellor's Department (1997) *Who Decides? Making Decisions on Behalf of Mentally Incapacitated Adults*. The Stationery Office, London.

9
The future

The current private contracted-out system of domiciliary or home care was mainly an outcome of paragraphs 3.4.1–3.6.3 in the 1989 White Paper *Caring for People*, and was, necessarily, relatively untried. Since then, the principle of contracting for services in general has been refined, and various services, such as the utilities, are evolving improved methods of conducting their affairs. This is commonly done in the light of failures or inefficiencies perceived since the initial bursts of activity.

However, the delivery of 'care' to the consumer's home has not been achieving the levels of success that might be the case with other services. Problems in funding override all other considerations, but there are also inherent problems in providing a private service hitherto untried in its scale, where the business risks so evenly balance the market demand. The high demand is very tempting for an entrepreneur, but the difficulties in meeting that demand can exceed the extent of that demand. Whereas setting up a nursing home in a locality undersupplied with such places has been seen as a more worthwhile gamble.

The demise of residential homes

But now, as we reach the end of the 1990s, statistics and surveys reveal that institutions are losing popularity to the concept of remaining in one's home as long as possible, with some assistance. Compared with running a residential home, which has established rules, timetables, staffing rotas, catering and laundering facilities on site, providing a domiciliary service has much greater demands on management. Management staff are more expensive, usually requiring benefits such as occupational pensions, occupational sick pay, paid holidays in excess of the statutory 3 weeks and intensive, costly training. One general manager used in a shift system, plus a number of care workers and nurses, can be deployed to run a residential home of 30–50 residents.

The same overall manager could run more than one home. New care workers can be trained initially by accompanying other trained ones. The important ratio is the number of care workers to residents. This is where staffing costs are critical.

In order to compare the two types of business, it is necessary to use the same units of turnover, which could only be hours, as using the number of residents in a residential home could not be paralleled in a domiciliary service. Although the property charges of a residential home, as well as catering and laundry, will enormously depress profitability, a general rule of thumb is to divide the turnover, in this case hours, by the number of staff, to obtain the cost and profitability of a business unit – an hour.

A home runs for 24 hours per day, 7 days per week. Thus 168 hours multiplied by the number of residents, in our example we will use 50, provides 8400 hours of care, which will be divided by the number of care staff.

Recruiting care workers for homes is generally much easier than recruiting care workers to work in the homes of individual clients, for many reasons. The financial limits of the business are determined by the physical bed space, and successful managers can open another home on another site or extend the existing one. Such capital investment presents enormous risks. And yet, from the business point of view, it still has the potential for a more secure profit, because the demands on management are known and are significantly less than the demands on the management of a proper professional domiciliary care service.

How does domiciliary care compare?

A domiciliary care service would be thriving on 8400 care hours per week, but the number of managerial staff required to provide what is in effect a one-to-one service would be much higher than for a residential home. A care worker in a home, looking after between three and five residents on average, may be paid at the same level as a care worker for a domiciliary agency, who will only be caring for one individual at a time. The staffing costs in a home decrease even further during the night.

Although the ancillary work in a home, such as catering and laundry, is a significant cost, it does not require such close management. Well-run homes will operate with a stable workforce, few changes and low-profile management.

Thus, the costs per hour of each type of business, taking into account the property charges, may show that a residential home bought a long time ago is a lesser risk than the alternative. But the price of property, the uneconomic fees paid by SSDs and the reluctance of private individuals to enter residential homes contribute to a changing picture.

If elderly and disabled people want improved domiciliary services, there must be some change in the manner of supply, if it is not going to be provided by the state. Professions have long been criticised for operating in their own interests and against the interests of the people who require their services. But businesses have no alternative to operating profitably. If the state is going to supply domiciliary care, whether as an integral service or contracted out to private organisations, there are still major logistical problems in the efficient servicing of localities within public spending limits.

Other Western economies

At this point, it is interesting to observe, albeit superficially, how some other Western economies facing the same demographic changes are addressing the demand for increased social care.

Germany

In Germany, the national sickness insurance scheme excluded long-term health- and social-care needs in old age. The ageing process was considered normal and not a medical problem. Many elderly people were obliged to use up their savings to pay for care until they became impoverished and so eligible to claim social assistance. But such financial help as was available was fragmented, and limited in its scope: 'In summary, the consequences of these very fragmented entitlements to the costs of long-term care were piecemeal care provision, a strong pull towards institutionalised care, catastrophic costs for older people needing long-term care and a lack of social security and social protection for informal carers'.[1] Provision for this care was through six welfare non-profit organisations who served particular social categories of people, appearing to form a 'cartel', and service standards were neither uniform nor imaginative.

Care insurance was seen as the solution, and in 1994, a mandatory scheme was implemented to cover the costs of 'care dependency'. This condition had to have national standards, and was measured according to the time taken for an assistant to enable the claimant to personal care, eating and mobility. Formal assessment is through a medical board, who make an assessment of 'care dependence' according to a grading system. Eligible claimants can obtain cash to pay for care or benefits in kind. Cash payments are much more popular than a formal care service, even though they are worth only half the cost of the formal care service. This cash is usually spent on the informal carers, and the monitoring of the quality of care given to the claimant by the informal carers is undertaken through periodic visits from a care provider of their choice. Organisations wishing to provide care are encouraged, and this includes individuals, all of whom must register with the organisations providing care insurance funds.

Problems with respect to co-ordination and lack of innovation still persist, 'but after four years of operation, the care insurance scheme has been judged to be successful'.[1] However, the long-term costs of this scheme are held as unsustainable.

Interestingly, the medical boards conducting the assessments have a duty to consider rehabilitation as part of the care dependency support systems.

Under the insurance scheme, care providers operate strictly capped budgets, index-linked to inflation. Costs are likely to rise, and there is little incentive for improvements in services, especially as the purchasers, the care insurance funds, make prospective agreements with the providers, tying them down to current costs: 'The care insurance funds have gained considerable power over the setting and regulation of prices ... in contrast, the regulation of standards of quality is weak'.[1]

There are no agreed guidelines for staffing levels of institutional care homes, and the standards within each agreement, locally controlled, are prone to variation. Home-care staff, however, are more regulated, and must have specific qualifications.

In conclusion, the pressure to contain costs has resulted in a closely specified, task-based service, with little prospect of co-ordination with other aspects of the health and welfare system.

The Netherlands

In The Netherlands, providing long-term care for elderly people has suffered from fragmentation of responsibility for the service, divisions between local and central government boundaries, and unresolved issues relating to providing care and cash benefits. However, there is considerably less distinction between health- and social-care services:

'Home nursing and home help services, nursing homes and residential care homes are treated equally within a single regulatory and financial framework'.[2] The basic elements of long-term care services are:

- institutional care funded jointly by the state through the national care fund and the client
- community-based services funded as above
- adapted and sheltered housing funded by social housing organisations and residential homes
- technical aids such as wheelchairs funded by local government
- social welfare services, funded through local government.

In the delivery and organisation of the health services for the whole population, there is a clear distinction between 'cure and care', and the health providers are funded by social health insurance for those falling below a threshold income, health insurance for civil servants and private health insurance schemes for those above the income threshold.

Long-term care has its own national fund, derived from tax-related premiums from all citizens and central government, but private insurance is playing an increasingly more significant role, as service charges based on factors including income levels have been introduced. Care services are provided by non-profit organisations which must comply with standards of quality. 'Increasingly, local, or regional providers of ... care are building joint ventures, and other alliances, and this is contributing to the emergence of an oligopolistic market'.[2] In response, the government is introducing 'benchmarking', 'which will control service providers' outputs, quality and prices through inter-provider comparisons of clearly defined "products"'.[2] Thus, there is an increasing realisation of the need for accountability and the need for cost-effectiveness, in spite of the relative success of the policy for publicly funded long-term care.

Personal budgets are part of a policy to experiment with care provision, on the basis that the present system is unresponsive and inflexible. It has proved successful, and the policy may be expanded. Applicants can spend their budget on care-related services in the home, and also to 'buy' from informal care-givers. Assessment for eligibility depends on the need, expressed in the number of hours of care a person might need, after taking into account what the family members will do. Reassessments are 6-monthly, and fees may be charged, depending on the income level. The budget is not held by the claimant *in toto*, but is partly controlled by an intermediary. This policy decision was taken in order to allay fears that the budgets would be spent in the unofficial labour market.

Private and public providers are constrained by requirements to comply with quality standards. These are measured by qualified personnel. Collective labour agreements for professional home helpers and nursing personnel in home care must be implemented.

To conclude, in spite of the freedom of the personal budget policy, consumers are still unable to influence the providers, and the government has introduced measures to create boards of consumer representatives. But the boards who make the assessments will be driven by the funding mechanisms, which will inevitably restrict financial resources.

Australia

The Australian system for funding long-term care has also suffered from fragmentation, again owing to the differing funding sources for acute healthcare and ongoing care. The political constitution has deeply affected the way in which health and social services are supplied. A central Australian or federal government is largely responsible for non-health care, but health or medical services are funded by State or Territory governments.

Legislation in the 1950s had the effect of excluding hospitals from the provision of long-term care for elderly people, and gave rise to an unprecedented growth in private nursing homes subsidised by the Commonwealth government. Government-funded community care services coexisted with this plethora of nursing homes, but for-profit providers did not receive government funding.

After considerable concern over the control of the provisions for elderly and disabled people, a new government in the 1980s introduced a co-ordinated long-term care system. Tighter control on funding was brought about, and a more general move towards care in the community and away from nursing homes began. 'As a result of these changes, a gradual shift in expenditure in favour of community took place. In the early 1980s, 11 dollars was spent on nursing homes and hostels for every 1 dollar spent on community care ... By 1991 this ratio had changed to 4.7 : 1.'[3] It could reach 3 : 1 by the year 2001.

The chief political question was which body was to be responsible for funding long-term care. Logically, the same organisations who funded medical care should also take over the budget for long-term care, but this issue, of enormous sensitivity, was left unchanged for fear of the cost implications.

Australia being a federation of states, there is no single system throughout the country. However, the current system is heavily dependent on hospitalisation, and post-acute care on the discharge of a patient tends to be central to methods of funding. Hospital staff hold budgets to purchase post-acute care, and appear to have the lead decision-making capacity. 'It is also argued that where community support services do exist, they do not offer the type or timeliness of support the hospital believes necessary; that they do not have the required level of skill; or that appropriate post-acute care services are outside the scope of the existing funding programmes for community care.'[3]

A number of trials are proposed in a drive for reform, and the introduction of competition within the care-provider system has also been discussed.

How is the current policy trend to be implemented?

The observed trend in neighbouring and similar economies is the change in policy towards driving health-related social care into the community and away from institutions. This is not without a significant bureaucratic cost, as well as the perennial conflict over the definitions of the limits of healthcare.

It is evident from the above that obstacles to providing efficient and consumer-sensitive domiciliary care are the classification of this service and the nature of its control – is it an extension of the health service, and so funded under the same principles as healthcare, or is it part of the welfare system which is available as a safety net to those who cannot provide for themselves? These questions must be answered in order that we can establish how the service is paid for – determining the levels of finance available.

From the point of view of the purchasers, both in the UK and elsewhere, care management is a constant theme, whether it is for post-acute hospital dischargees or for those electing not to move into a residential home but remain in their own property and rely on an external provider of care services to call on a regular basis.

Returning to discussion of the UK system, the present government set up a Royal Commission to examine the way in which long-term care could be funded. In its report in March 1999, *With Respect to Old Age:*

Long Term Care – Rights and Responsibilities, criticising the unfairness of the present system, there was a majority decision and additional comments from two members who dissented from the final recomendations. The overall opinion in the majority report was that residential care was often sought by the professionals as the preferred alternative, even if it did not concur with the wishes of the individual. In considering the the distribution of costs, it proposed that all nursing and personal care should be paid for by the state through general taxation, and that a National Care Commission should be put in place to monitor longitudinal trends such as demography and spending, to provide transparency and accountability, and to set rates and standards for home personal care. Given sufficient powers to make it truly effective, this would put the control of such personal care outside the health service and may quell the debate over what is and is not healthcare. The minority report, opposing the recommendation for free personal care, proposed a greater development of community or domiciliary care and more support for the voluntary carers. The provision of care would still depend on an assessment of needs, and it is difficult to speculate how much choice would be available.

It is anticipated that the government will publish its own proposals within a year, but the cost implications of the Commission's recommendations have not gone unnoticed. The Commission itself admitted to a 'funnel of doubt' with respect to the forecast of its costings.

Whether the funding is through the state or through an insurance fund, a managed package of care has to be arranged by someone. Some of the countries described above have set up elaborate boards of control, assessment and screening units, which all require considerable investment in human resources, not to mention the constant policy dichotomy related to funding criteria. This piecemeal, individualised examination of every individual's health-related social needs, not just once, but periodically, will exceed the demands on managerial staff previously devoted to the discrete long-term care of the client group. An analogous comparison might be the effort required to manufacture a single design repeatedly and the effort required to custom design every item for the customers.

The management of care

Increasingly, private individuals and recipients of state grants are able to decide for themselves, and as Caroline Glendinning comments, 'behaving as a "consumer" of long-term care services requires a degree of literacy, confidence and competence'.[4]

The current method of deploying personnel for home-care social services is extremely wasteful of human and other resources. The requirements of businesses to cover large areas, and the consequential need for the care workers to travel distances, incurs extra costs. The local geographical nature of the demand calls for the supply to be determined on the same basis. In order to reduce such problems, there is much talk of partnership between social services and the healthcare departments, as well as partnership between state-funded institutions and the private sector.

The sheer wastefulness of the present system, coupled with increasing demand for home care, should engender new thinking on the methods of supplying the service. The current situation, where many people who want work, are willing to do the work and are able to do the work, but simply do not have the high mobility that the erratic demand requires, is a less than efficient use of such valuable resources and goodwill. Furthermore, such people are deprived of a steady source of income on which they can depend and develop their own independence.

Another problem is that it is unlikely that such a service will ever become a profitable one for private organisations, in spite of the demand, as statutory purchasers have tight budgets, and the highly vocal demand for children's services means that other social services tend to have a lower priority. Furthermore, the majority of private clients will be disinclined to pay higher rates for a service that they have been getting cheaply hitherto.

The multiple requirements of the different branches of health and social care can result in what appears occasionally to be an unco-ordinated succession of staff calling at the home of a service user, client or patient. Such poor co-ordination points to a lack of organisation in the deployment of scant resources, especially when large numbers of qualified, and possibly well-paid, staff have to spend many hours of the working day travelling in their cars, calling at the homes of clients/patients.

If the delivery of services to the home of the recipient is the 'holy grail', then it may be useful to consider what incentives would be required to achieve the outcome. The greatest blight on the project is the insufficiency of staff to provide the care services, and it may be necessary to ask why this is so and if solutions can be found.

Using an outcomes approach, where an organisation is contracted to provide holistic care for service users, considered by some to have more long-term benefit, brings difficulties when more than one organisation is attending to one client. How can the competence and success of a single organisation at achieving the goals be assessed if one is measuring the state of well being of the service user? Furthermore, the provision of 'holistic' care would necessitate a relationship of trust, commonly found in the medical and alternative therapies. Although contracting relationships do not exclude mutuality and trust, that is not their general use and purpose, and so creating a holistic, outcomes-based deployment of resources requires a different approach.

An alternative approach could be a partnership. A partnership is a contract between individuals or organisations in which the risks and benefits are more transparent than in a contract to supply, and are taken into account in creating the many terms within the partnership agreement. It is a method of determining how each of the parties in the relationship will act and react in given circumstances, and when new and unforeseen circumstances arise provides for a method of resolution while the primary, ongoing activities continue uninterrupted. It is a relationship that bridges the gap of mutual mistrust in the pursuit of a single set of goals. In a range of transactional relationships, it is somewhere between contracting for supply and total merger or integration.

Possible reconfigurations

Scenario one: locality

The SSD divides the local authority area into sectors, not unlike the way in which areas for family services GPs are defined, and requires private or not-for-profit organisations to provide the care services for each sector. It is assumed that the funding criteria are unchanged from the present system, where eligibility for SSD-funded care depends on the personal wealth of the individual. This would enable the care provider or agency to employ staff on a proper footing, with regular hours and steady incomes, and, most advantageous of all, the majority of travelling could be done on foot. In this way, more people who might otherwise do voluntary work may be attracted to help a neighbour. The greatest use is made of the spare time of adults, as well as providing work for those who find caring an enjoyable form of employment.

Scenario two: goods and services

The SSDs request large, well-known or high-street organisations to bid for the appropriate servicing of specific localities, whose care needs have already been mapped, in order to fix a funding limit. The organisation must provide all necessary social-care services, and is free to sell to the residents any goods, e.g. domestic appliances, mobility appliances, incontinence aids, safety appliances, toiletries and so forth. Where the value of transactions could be more than the cost of the care service alone, and so profitability is more of a possibility, then high-street organisations, such as a pharmacists, would have incentives to train staff and ensure a high quality of home caring. Such services may require monitoring to ensure that exploitation of vulnerable people is excluded.

Scenario three: the care community

The SSDs and health authorities in the shape of the new primary care groups jointly divide the area into sectors and provide a home-care service, which is free to those who, on the basis of means testing, need not pay, but for those who have means, the true cost is charged. The advantage to the health services here is that they can be involved not only in the manner of hospital discharges, but also in the training and monitoring of the effectiveness of the service. A closer relationship between institutional and domiciliary services can be sought on a much more localised basis.

Scenario four: outreach

Local nursing homes are invited to bid for providing a domiciliary service to the locality in which they are situated, and can also provide respite periods for individuals. This system is already in existence, but the lack of a geographical boundary means that many requests for domiciliary care must be declined, as the organising home cannot find a suitable care worker in the location of the client or service user.

Scenario five: community co-operative

On the basis that many individuals are in receipt of grants to enable them to purchase care provision on the open market, there should be a pool of potential care workers available to do the work. Rather than have the transaction brokered by an agency, both parties could empower themselves if local training organisations could provide the appropriate training for such potential care workers, after which the trained care worker could register with the relevant benefits agency dispensing the grants. Any potential care consumer in receipt of a grant could be provided with the register and elect to contract with their own care worker. The training organisation could be in a position to provide references and further or ongoing training. Here, the critical aspect is to keep the spread of the localities to a very limited size and so decrease the probability of strangers on the scene, whose past history cannot be verified.

Conclusion

The main principle, which ought to apply to any provider of care services, is that the outcomes are clarified. Service-level agreements are useful, detailed guides about how a service ought to be undertaken, but if the objectives of the service are known, then these also should be included in the contracts. Without this ultimate 'purpose', the providers under contract are merely subcontractors, and their behaviour will resemble that of subcontractors in general, whose main function is usually compliance, because no more is required of them. A true partnership involves sharing of business goals, risk, burden and profitability. If SSDs intend to make use of the private, for-profit sector, then contracts should not be drawn so tightly as to eliminate any possibility of profit, giving rise to bad employment practices.

Unless there is a pool of kindly citizens who are prepared to work within people's homes for a large part of the day – or night – the private home-care sector will not thrive. The individuals who are prepared to do such heroic work are at least deserving of a decent and steady income. The need for a constant and reliable source of income is of greater priority than a high income. In human resource terms, the workers are the most valuable commodity in the provision of community care, and their needs will be just as relevant as those of the client group.

References

1 Schunk M (1998) The social insurance model of care for older people in Germany. In: C Glendinning (ed.) *Rights and Realities: Comparing New Developments in Long Term Care for Older People*. The Policy Press, Bristol.

2 Coolen J and Weekers S (1998) Long-term care in The Netherlands: public funding and private provision within a universalistic welfare state. In: C Glendinning (ed.) *Rights and Realities: Comparing New Developments in Long Term Care for Older People*. The Policy Press, Bristol.

3 Fine M (1998) Acute and continuing care for older people in Australia: contesting new balances of care. In: C Glendinning (ed.) *Rights and Realities: Comparing New Developments in Long Term Care for Older People*. The Policy Press, Bristol.

4 Glendinning C (1998) Conclusions: learning from abroad. In: C Glendinning (ed.) *Rights and Realities: Comparing New Developments in Long Term Care for Older People*, p. 137. The Policy Press, Bristol.

Appendix

The Hon Secretary
Age Concern
Astral House
1268 London Road
London SW1 4ER

The Hon Secretary
Alzheimer's Disease Society
Gordon House
10 Greencoat Place
London SW1P 1PH

The Hon Secretary
Carers National Association
20–25 Glasshouse Yard
London EC14 4JS

Independent Financial Advice Bureau
549 Green Lanes
Haringay
London N8 0RQ

The Hon Secretary
Insurance Ombudsman
City Gate One
135 Park Street
London SE1 9EA

The Hon Secretary
The Personal Investment Authority
1 Canada Square
Canary Wharf
London E14 5AZ

The Hon Secretary
UKHCA
42b Banstead Road
Carshalton Beeches
Surrey SM5 3NW

The Hon Secretary
NCVO
Regent's Wharf
8 All Saints Road
London N1 9RL

Index